Paraplegia

PARAPLEGIA
A handbook of practical care and advice

MICHAEL A. ROGERS

With a Foreword by
the Right Honourable
Baroness Masham of Ilton
Countess of Swinton

FABER AND FABER
London   Boston

First published in 1978
by Faber and Faber Limited
3 Queen Square London WC1N 3AU
Printed in Great Britain by
Butler & Tanner Ltd
Frome and London

CONDITIONS OF SALE

British Library Cataloguing in Publication Data

Rogers, Michael A
Paraplegia.
1. Paralytics – Care and treatment
I. Title
362.1'9'6837   HV3011

ISBN 0–571–11209–9
ISBN 0–571–11208–0   Pbk

with love and gratitude,
I dedicate this book
to my wife, ELIZABETH,
without whose constant support
it would not have been written

Contents

Illustrations

Foreword

Michael Rogers was born in 1937 and educated at Caldicott School, Farnham Common and Trent College, Nottingham. He served for three years in the Royal Electrical and Mechanical Engineers (R.E.M.E.) spending two years in Cyprus attached to the Royal Horse Guards where he was responsible for maintenance of all escort transport at Government House, Nicosia. After he was discharged from the Army in 1958 Michael established a plant machinery business. In 1960 he contracted an unknown virus infection of the spinal cord which left him paralysed below the shoulders, thus making him a tetraplegic with all four limbs paralysed.

Michael spent 18 months in a London teaching hospital – where he developed many of the known complications in paraplegia; pressure sores, contractures of the limbs, kidney and bladder stones, and chest complications. He was finally transferred to the spinal unit at Stoke Mandeville Hospital in a serious condition. Three and a half years were spent correcting the complications. He was finally discharged in 1965 after spending nearly five years in hospitals.

Michael Rogers cares about his fellow paraplegics and tetraplegics; and for this reason he decided to write this book which he hopes will help to prevent some of the suffering he had experienced. He knows as I know, that there is still much lack of knowledge in dealing with the severely paralysed.

Michael is a most meticulous person and has taken several years researching the material for this book. He knows that to keep fit as a para or tetraplegic one has to live an organized life keeping to a sensible routine. To neglect one's daily routine as a paralysed person puts one at great risk.

Michael sets out very clearly in this book guidelines which should be helpful to many people who may be looking after a paralysed person or who may be paralysed themselves. It is impossible to really know the inner struggles and feelings and the attitudes to life from a paralysed person's point of view unless one has had first hand experience.

Despite this catastrophic illness, Michael has managed to pick up the threads of life. He is married to Elizabeth, now a nursing officer on a spinal unit, and they live in a very homely attractive house. For relaxation Michael paints in oils with brushes held in his teeth. He has helped with a two-year research project on employment for tetraplegics and he is a very active member of the Spinal Injuries Association.

With shortage of money in our National Health Service the correct treatment of paraplegia is vital not only to save suffering but also to save resources and extra time spent in hospital putting right the wrongs of maltreatment, be it due to hospital or home care.

I hope Michael's book will help to further the understanding of paraplegia, both for families and friends, as well as for all members of the health caring team.

SUSAN MASHAM
House of Lords 1978

Author's Preface

During the past seventeen years as a tetraplegic, I have met many people involved directly and indirectly with those who have suffered spinal cord injuries resulting in paraplegia or tetraplegia. Many of these people, particularly the close relatives and at a later stage of their treatment the patients themselves, have expressed difficulties in finding a concise practical publication about spinal injuries. They have looked for something which can be clearly understood by those who have never heard of the existence of the spinal cord and the many problems connected with its damage.

The National Spinal Injuries Centre at Stoke Mandeville hospital was founded in 1944 by Sir Ludwig Guttmann, and since then few books have been written about paraplegia essentially for the benefit of patients and their relatives. I am not over-looking two commendable books *Understanding Paraplegia* by Dr J. J. Walsh and the Spinal Injuries Association publication *so you're paralysed* written by Bernadette Fallon. Despite their qualities and excellent content, both books still leave many questions unanswered. There is also a great deal of advice, guidance and information as yet unpublished. With this in mind and many pleas for additional facts ringing in my ears I have written this book. I believe it to be the first comprehensive production prepared and set out specifically for patients and their relatives.

I have received help and guidance on technical matters from a spinal injuries specialist and also from my wife who is the nursing officer at the Spinal Injuries Centre, Stoke Mandeville Hospital.

In many chapters I have been blunt and frank, particularly regarding sexual functions. I know that many people are shy to talk about the subject, including some doctors and nurses, and especially those employed outside specialized spinal injury centres. With modern methods of treatment, patients now spend less time in hospital and when discharged are not always mentally adjusted to the many problems that will remain with them for the rest of their lives.

Before the National Spinal Injuries Centre was founded, many paraplegics and even more tetraplegics, failed to survive. This was because the necessary medical treatment and nursing care was not fully understood. Consequently, a person suffering a spinal cord injury often received inadequate treatment in some corner of a general hospital ward, with minimal chances of survival. Today the situation is vastly different; new techniques have evolved, research has progressed and knowledge gained through the world's spinal injuries centres, has completely changed the picture. Patients treated by modern methods in specialized centres and later discharged, can look forward to a normal lifespan, providing correct medical supervision continues. Where circumstances allow, the paraplegic or tetraplegic can do a rewarding job of work. Indeed, it has often been found that disabled people are more highly motivated towards work than they were before their injury.

One fact cannot be overlooked. In most cases of traumatic injury, the paralysis, varying in degree according to the extent and site of the actual injury, is permanent. Patients will have to learn a new way of living if they are to survive and enjoy a worthwhile existence.

During the early days of treatment following a spinal cord injury many things will appear to be utterly hopeless to the patient. A feeling of despondency will inevitably set in and the outlook for the future will seem bleak. This is the time when help and understanding from the medical and paramedical staff is all important. Vital, too, is comfort and re-assurance from relatives who will have been **correctly** briefed, for they can play an essential part in helping patients rediscover life and themselves.

The major prerequisite for success is that a patient fully understands the new situation; which will include a sound, comprehensive knowledge of the medical condition, with all its implications and demands. From the outset, it cannot be over emphasized to patients that they must be prepared to maintain a high standard of vigilance throughout their lives to ensure that their new style of living is strictly adhered to, and that methods laid down by medical staff are correctly maintained at all times.

Acknowledgements

In the writing of this book I have been indebted to many people – not least to numerous fellow paraplegics who have offered much encouragement.

Firstly I would like to thank Baroness Masham for kindly writing the Foreword and for her encouragement at all times.

I would particularly like to thank Jack Hill, the South Coast correspondent of the *Daily Express*, and Dennis Mimmack of Elstree, Hertfordshire.

To Mr I. M. Nuseibeh, FRCS, Consultant Surgeon in Spinal Injuries, Stoke Mandeville Hospital, my grateful thanks not only for vetting the medical details but also for his constant support.

I am grateful to Mrs Audrey Besterman and Helen Tory for the illustrations and to Derek Standen for the photographs.

The chapter on transport owes much to the marvellous co-operation of the Ford Motor Company of Britain Ltd., Brentwood, Essex, who went to endless trouble to provide information. Similarly the Joint Committee on Mobility for the Disabled, the Disabled Drivers Association and the Disabled Drivers Motor Club were all most helpful and I am grateful to them.

Her Majesty's Stationery Office has given permission for the publishing of the extract from the Chronically Sick and Disabled Persons Act 1970.

Finally, I thank Faber and Faber for their help and advice at all times in the production of this book.

Definitions

A paraplegic is a person with paralysis involving the lower limbs. Part or the whole of the trunk may also be paralysed.

A tetraplegic is a person with paralysis involving all four limbs. The whole trunk may also be paralysed.

Throughout this book, reference made to a paraplegic will include the tetraplegic, unless otherwise stated.

1

Some Psychological Aspects
of Paralysis

Following the admission to hospital of a spinal injury patient, close relatives will find themselves in a state of mental turmoil when they are told that their loved one is paralysed. The initial reaction is one of shock in a world of strange words, new faces, hospital equipment and disabled people in varying stages of treatment. Later, a patient or next-of-kin will want to know why paralysis has been caused.

Why does a person become paralysed when their spine is broken? A very good question; for some people do break their spines without becoming paralysed. This is because in their cases the spinal cord, made up of thousands of nerve fibres linking the brain with various parts of the body, has not been damaged despite the fractured vertebrae of the spinal column. Paralysis occurs whenever those minute nerve fibres have been damaged or broken during the spinal accident, as is explained in detail in the next chapter.

The next question to be asked is: will the patient recover? This is a difficult one for doctors to answer immediately. A period of time, known as the period of 'spinal shock' must elapse to allow the spinal cord to recover from the shock of injury. This period can take eight or more weeks. For the patient, family and friends it is a time of tension, anxiety and heartache. To help people over this period, it is important to have a little understanding of some of the psychological aspects of paralysis.

According to the *Oxford Dictionary*, psychology is the study of the human soul or mind. Therefore the psychological effect of paralysis is just another way of saying what goes on in the minds of patients and their families and friends. During the very early stages after becoming paralysed, whether the cause was traumatic, such as a motor car or diving accident, or non-traumatic, such as an illness, I think it is fair to say that the average patient is far too bewildered and frightened as well as too ill, to think clearly about what has happened to him. He will give little thought to the fact that he is unable to move or feel certain parts of his body.

On admission to hospital, complete and utter trust is instinctively placed in the hands of the medical and nursing professions and subconsciously the patient feels that all will be well. After a day or two, most patients begin to feel a little better. Mental confusion subsides and the mind starts to recover its original pattern of thinking. But often a sense of panic is experienced at this stage and desperate questions fill the head. 'What has happened to me?' 'Why can't I feel or move?' 'Why can't I feel my bladder and bowels?' Also the embarrassment and humiliation of being physically exposed every few hours for turns and medical procedures, can be devastating.

Patients will begin to take notice of their surroundings, observe other patients in wheelchairs and listen to endless conversations between patients and staff about paraplegia, its problems and their day-to-day progress. At this stage many patients experience intense psychological disturbances and will, for varying periods of time, require all the love, care and understanding that can possibly be given.

Similarly, close relatives will be suffering the same feelings, possibly more so, for they will have been told right from the start how serious the situation is for their loved one. Unfortunately there is no quick and simple answer to the heartaches that must inevitably follow. There are no wonder or miracle drugs to put everything right. The process of psychological adjustment is slow and only time can heal the hurt mind successfully. To help relatives through this desperate and traumatic period, it is essential they understand the various stages of paraplegia. It is even more important that relatives appreciate and understand their loved one's feelings and reactions to this strange new world.

The natural reaction of most patients is to wonder, 'Why me?' 'What have I done to deserve this?' Many dispel their emotions by crying or cursing and swearing at everybody and everything in sight. Some will pray endlessly, trying to find an answer and rid their minds about the reality of their condition. Close relatives, wives, husbands, mothers, fathers, brothers, and sisters, boy or girl friends are those most likely to receive the brunt of this abuse. It is human nature to hurt those you love most. Ward staff will get it next; nurses, orderlies, physiotherapists; even the doctors. For nothing anybody does can be right at this stage and it seems there is nothing anybody can do to make it right.

This can be a most distressing time for relatives. No matter what they say or do, they are quite unable to alter the situation.

There are many things they *can* do to help at the hospital bedside; things that make the patient feel better at this most distressing and emotionally exhausting period. I list a few for guidance:

Try hard to maintain your natural normal everyday self. Do not suddenly adopt a different personality, for this will disturb and worry the patient. Spend as much time at the bedside as possible, doing the little things that the patient may ask you to do. Avoid being over-protective or too possessive. Do not be over-anxious to help, as this only emphasizes the limitations of the patient.

It is best for relatives to involve themselves with the medical procedures taking place, by questioning doctors, nurses, physiotherapists and other members of staff. This helps the patient appreciate that his relatives are interested in learning about his condition.

Medical experts in the field of spinal injury and its attendant psychology, recognize the established fact that many patients suddenly become unusually aggressive at this stage. It can be most disturbing, and relatives need to understand that aggression during this period is far better than mere apathy. It is known as 'reactionary aggression' and is a good sign. Aggressive patients, although sometimes abrasive and abusive, have 'got fight'. The mentally apathetic succumb far too easily and will have greater difficulty in rehabilitating to their new life-style.

During this initial period and for some time to follow, patients will be faced with the most soul-destroying and distressing situations imaginable. If a maximum effort is not made by all concerned to lessen these unusual and embarrassing situations, further psychological disturbances may follow. This is often more apparent in females, who may have led more sheltered physical lives than men.

It is necessary for patients to spend considerable periods of time completely naked. Bedclothes will be removed for washing, bowel management, catheter drill, dressings, turns, physiotherapy treatment and other regular examinations. During these procedures screens should be drawn around the beds. Staff sometimes forget this, or fail to close curtains tightly together, leaving patients to suffer unnecessary embarrassment of exposure. This can only retard mental adjustment. Relatives and patients can therefore help each other by insisting on a high standard of privacy.

One would think that the psychological effect on a person losing the use of all four limbs is greater than on a person losing his legs alone. Yet this is not always the case. It is all relative to the individual and it is wrong to compare degrees of reaction.

Patients who have lost the use of their legs, will lie in bed thinking of obvious things they can no longer do; like dancing, climbing, walking, football, and getting about the house and garden. At first they will give no thought to the many things that they **can** do. Patients with the loss of all four limbs will *think* about these aspects, but will be more concerned with scratching their noses, combing hair, washing, brushing teeth, feeding themselves or even holding the hands of close friends or relatives.

All will naturally wonder about their sexual function, or the loss of it. But at this early stage they will ask nothing, for they will not know what to ask. This subject is dealt with comprehensively in Chapter 6.

During the following weeks, the days will be filled with a tiresome but vital combination of routine treatments. There will be doctors' rounds; intermittent catheterisations to empty the bladder; the endless three or four hourly turns day and night to prevent pressure sores. Daily physiotherapy in the form of passive and some active movements of limbs to keep joints mobile and the non-paralysed muscles active, and occupational therapy to maintain and strengthen existing movements, as well as keeping the mind alert. Throughout this routine treatment, the basic principles of future care become increasingly apparent. So at last when the stage of spinal shock has passed, the dreaded question has finally to be asked: 'Doctor, am I going to recover any more?' This is a problem for doctors. Exactly when and how they should answer this question is debatable. Obviously the patient's general condition has to be considered. I would plead that doctors who read this book, should be as certain as possible before answering this question. Please tell the truth; but with great tact, and with comforting words and reassurance regarding the future.

Although most patients will subconsciously know the answer before asking, final condemnation to a wheelchair is quite catastrophic.

Let nobody underestimate the psychological and physical effect of being told that you will never walk again; or the even worse effect of being told that you will never use your hands again. It can only be likened to a judge passing a life sentence.

No matter how distressing this might be, the truth is better than telling a patient that he will be 'fine tomorrow'. For tomorrow never comes and the long term depressive effect will be greater if the truth is withheld. Many patients choose to avoid asking if they will recover. This is either in the hope that they will, or from a fear of what they might learn. In these circumstances I believe it is the doctor's duty to make the situation perfectly clear and to reiterate the truth more than once. For some patients will say many months later that they were never told.

No matter how tactfully patients are told that they will never walk or use their limbs again, most will initially wish they were dead and out of it. There seems so little left in life. This is a perfectly normal and understandable reaction and one that is usually followed by prolonged bouts of depression mixed with aggressive outbursts. The most satisfactory method of dealing with this depression is by diversional therapy. This means anything that will keep the mind occupied – and such therapy should be applied by all members of staff as well as by friends and relations during visits.

Nursing staff should talk about outside interests while carrying out routine nursing procedures. Doctors can help by continued daily visits, even if there is nothing medically necessary for them to do. Physiotherapists must explain the aims of the treatment they are providing, in order to gain the patient's interest. The occupational therapist can provide practical work, not only in the form of diversional therapy, but also to strengthen and maintain existing movements. This is not always easy with tetraplegics, who may have limited movements. Friends and relatives can best help by visiting as often as possible and talking of day-to-day matters. Relatives should also seek advice from experienced hospital staff about the patient's domestic future, so that blunt questions can be answered truthfully. This will all help to gently ease a patient's mind back into normal routine thinking.

No matter how hard medical, nursing, and paramedical staff work to relieve depression, they will not succeed unless the patient fights tremendously hard himself to overcome this despairing state of mind.

Paraplegics can do a great deal to help themselves but tetraplegics will find it harder. Both paraplegics and tetraplegics should start by making an extra effort to smile, talk and be cheerful to staff and relatives. This is not as easy as it sounds. It will require maximum willpower, but once a start has been made, cheerfulness and optimism will come more naturally.

Reading is an excellent method of keeping the mind occupied. Bookrests are available in hospital, together with a large selection of books. Where difficulty is experienced in turning pages or holding a book, there is a 'talking book' service. Books are recorded on tape and all one has to do is wear a set of headphones and listen. This is easy, for it requires no physical effort and is a wonderful method of occupying the mind. Television and radio provide relaxation and most hospital beds are fitted with headphones that can be switched to any station or channel required.

It is so easy to lie in bed just counting spots on the ceiling and allowing the mind to wander and sleep. Beware! The longer this is done, the longer it will take to recover psychologically later on.

The majority of patients have domestic problems of one kind or another: hire purchase on a car; mortgage repayments; employment problems and schooling their children just to mention a few. These problems are typical of the many things that patients turn over in their minds as they lie in bed. Coupled with the added worries of paraplegia, both immediate and still to come, these domestic difficulties are often amplified or even invented.

I realize it is so easy to say don't worry, particularly where there may indeed be real problems. But worry really is the key to the whole situation. Try not to worry in advance. Take each day as it comes and close the mind to all future problems for the time being. By doing this, the mind is left clear to concentrate on a maximum effort towards rehabilitation. Finally, all those problems often turn out to be not half as bad as anticipated!

To help surmount this crucial period, patients can enlist the help of the hospital's social worker whose job it is to take over such domestic worries. At a later stage the social worker should be able to help and advise on most domestic problems, including housing, insurance claims, transport and employment. Many social workers have had many years' experience in dealing with the numerous social and domestic problems associated with paraplegia, and patients who find they cannot cope should bear this in mind.

Between 2 and 4 months from the time of injury is the usual

time taken for fractured bones to heal and for the spinal cord to recover from its injury and shock. Then the majority of patients will be ready to get up in a wheelchair. At this stage it is essential that those who have not been fortunate enough to recover from paralysis, must learn more about their physical condition, their limitations and how their body is affected. A simple explanation of their condition and how to cope with it is all that is required.

It does, however, need to be clearly understood and accepted philosophically, that as a paraplegic and particularly as a tetraplegic, life will be different in many ways from now on, and a new pattern of living has to be evolved.

2

Know Your Paralysis

ANATOMICAL UNDERSTANDING

The first thing patients need to learn is exactly what has happened to them. It is useless thinking that because the neck or back has been broken and paralysis has resulted, there is no further need to be concerned about the injury or its cause and effects. To survive successfully, patients must understand why there is paralysis and how the body reacts to it. The parts of the body stricken without feeling or movement are by no means dead and need to be looked after very carefully.

If the brain is thought of as a central power house or information centre, then it becomes easier for a patient to understand why it is that he becomes paralysed when his spine is broken. Messages are received in the brain in the form of electrical impulses, whenever a physical action is required. If this line of communication is broken, then there can be no response.

The impulses from the brain reach the muscles via the spinal cord. The spinal cord is made up of thousands of tiny nerve fibres, like fine wires, each about 45cm (18in) long. The cord is about the diameter of a man's little finger; this vulnerable cord is situated in the centre of the tough bony vertebral column for protection. The vertebral column is the spine; and inside the spine the cord is surrounded by fluid for further protection. It is nature's own form of armour plating.

The vertebral column is constructed of many segments or vertebrae, over thirty; each separated by discs of gristle, which form pads and shock absorbers that permit smooth bending of the spine. When the spine is broken the cord may be damaged; and when this happens, messages from the brain to parts of the body that lie below the site of injury are unable to get through. Some injuries are termed 'complete lesions' whilst others are 'incomplete lesions'. This is simply a way of defining whether the cord has been wholly or partly damaged. When partly damaged there may be partial sensation or movement below the point of injury. A complete lesion will allow no movement or sensation below the site of injury (Fig. 2/1).

Quite often a newly injured person will initially appear to have a complete lesion. After varying periods of time, as the spinal cord recovers from shock, swelling and bruising, sensation and movement begin to return and some patients make total recoveries. Nerves of the spinal cord cannot be repaired or replaced. For reasons not yet fully understood to medical science, nerves of the spinal cord will not grow together once they are broken.

Doctors and scientists are researching into this problem and may one day find an answer. Meanwhile research has been and is being conducted into the best possible methods of looking after people who have sustained spinal cord injuries.

To estimate how much of the body is affected by a spinal cord injury, medical experts have to perform a detailed examination. The severity of paralysis is dependent on which sections of the vertebral column and spinal cord were damaged during the accident or illness.

The vertebral column is divided into five groups of vertebrae as follows:

cervical vertebrae – 7
thoracic vertebrae – 12
lumbar vertebrae – 5
sacral vertebrae – 5
coccygeal vertebrae – 4
(sacral and coccygeal vertebrae are fused together and form the base of the spinal column).

The spinal cord running down through the vertebral column,

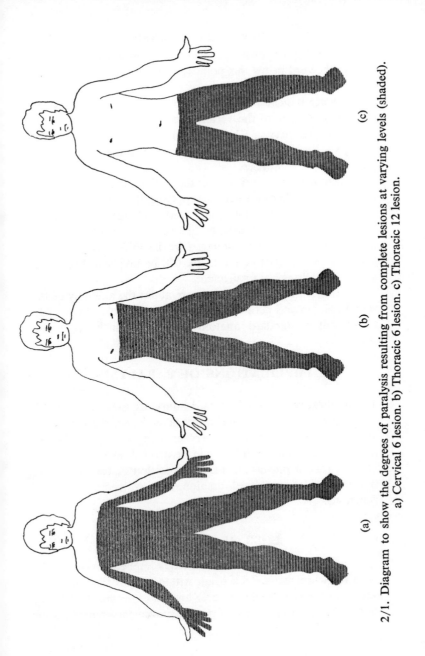

2/1. Diagram to show the degrees of paralysis resulting from complete lesions at varying levels (shaded). a) Cervical 6 lesion. b) Thoracic 6 lesion. c) Thoracic 12 lesion.

(a)
(b)
(c)

usually finishes opposite the second lumbar vertebra. Nerves leaving the cord below this point form what is called the cauda equina.

There are bunches of nerves, between the vertebrae, which emerge either side of the vertebral column, and are known as the peripheral nerves. They carry messages to and from the brain, via the spinal cord, to various parts of the body such as the skin and the muscles.

Most spinal cord injuries affect the bladder, bowels and sexual organs. This is because nerves supplying these functions stem from the lower end of the spinal cord. Damage to the cord in the cervical region, will usually involve hands, arms, trunk and legs. Where the cord is damaged in the mid-thoracic region, lower limbs and part of the trunk will be involved, but hands and arms will remain unaffected.

For those who wish to learn more about the anatomy of the spinal column and peripheral nerve roots, I would advise them to consult a standard anatomy textbook, such as *Gray's Anatomy*.

IMPLICATIONS OF PARALYSIS

The implications of a spinal cord injury are many and varied. Some very complex physical changes take place that are unnecessary for a patient to study, while other changes are more obvious and easily understood. These can be divided into several main groups: loss of movement, loss of sensation or feeling, loss of normal bladder and bowel function, and involvement of sexual functions.

LOSS OF MOVEMENT

Loss of movement is the most obvious implication, hence the need for wheelchairs. As a result within a short time of injury, wastage of muscle bulk can occur and limbs become thin. Daily physiotherapy, in the form of passive movements, must be given to all paralysed limbs, or joints will become stiff and tendons and muscles will shrink. Physiotherapy is most important in the early stages of hospital treatment to prevent stiffness and contractures, for any recovery of muscle power will be hampered by short, tight tendons and stiff joints. Electrotherapy is sometimes given to maintain specific muscle bulk, usually where recovery is evident. Its application to the whole of a paralysed body is totally impracticable.

Limbs not used for a number of years will obviously change in character. As well as muscle wastage, tendons will shorten and bones will decalcify and become brittle. This is known as osteoporosis, and is due to lack of weight-bearing and muscle pull. Regular standing under the instruction of a physiotherapist will reduce bone wastage. So will the taking of as much active exercise as possible (see p. 80). It is vital for children to stand as often and for as long as possible, under the instruction of their doctor, because without weight-bearing limbs will fail to grow normally.

Many patients develop spasms in their limbs. These are involuntary, jerky contractions of muscles, caused by over-active reflex movements due to damage of the spinal cord. Sometimes spasms have their advantages, including the maintenance of muscle tone, blood circulation and blood pressure. Remember, spasms can cause violent, involuntary movements of limbs and throw patients off balance. The first signs of spasticity occur at varying periods after injury and must not be interpreted as a sign of recovery. Physiotherapy and hydrotherapy together with good nursing care will reduce spasms. Surgical treatment is sometimes required in extreme cases; and this will be determined by the spinal specialist.

LOSS OF SENSATION

Sensation loss is probably the main factor in the many complications associated with paralysis. Without feeling or sensation there is no normal warning when bladder or bowels are full.

Sexual functions also depend largely on sensation. I will deal with both these aspects separately.

Consider what other problems can arise during the course of a normal day, where there is loss of sensation. There is a danger in summer that paralysed parts of the body may be sunburnt. This is best avoided by not sitting in direct sunlight on very hot days, by wearing a suitable hat and covering those parts without feeling.

In winter the need for extra heat often results in severe burns, which can be caused by sitting too close to open fires, against radiators or hot pipes. Hot water bottles should **never** be used. Electric blankets, both the over and under types, can cause burns and must **never** be used. Scalding from hot baths, hot drinks and from cooking accidents are other obvious dangers. Injury may occur from an accidental and trivial knock.

A combination of cold weather, loss of feeling and reduced circulation can result in frostbite on cold days. **Always cover** exposed limbs if you are going out when temperatures are low. If you are feeling cold, put on extra clothes or wrap up snugly in a blanket. It is far safer than sitting on top of a fire.

Sensation loss conceals pain which is a warning of possible complications. This makes a doctor's job of diagnosing internal problems more difficult. Patients must maintain constant and vigilant interest in themselves. This will include remembering what you have eaten, or drunk, as well as the drugs you may have taken, also the appearance of stools and urine. Where there is any alteration from your normal, you should tell your doctor without delay.

HEAT REGULATION

In cervical and high thoracic lesions, particularly in complete lesions, there will be involvement of the body temperature mechanism. On very hot days the blood temperature can easily increase. The opposite occurs in extreme cold. Most patients will have heard how elderly people suffer from 'hypothermia' or excess cold, and 'hyperthermia' or excess heat. The same applies to the paralysed, but from a different cause.

The body temperature mechanism is very complex. It can be more easily understood by thinking of the many things within the human body that happen involuntarily. A good example is 'goose flesh' the erection of little hairs on the skin surface, often triggered by a sudden flow of cold air. The regulation of the body temperature is similarly outside our control. The exertion of energy by physical movement or just sitting in hot sunshine causes skin and blood to increase in temperature. Several things occur to compensate for this. Sweat glands produce moisture on the skin surface, and this evaporates and takes away body heat. Circulation is increased forcing more blood to the skin's surface where it is cooled and thereby reduces blood temperature. These two reactions to heat occur automatically in an able-bodied person. The situation is different for the paraplegic.

The heat-regulating centre is situated in the brain, and with the aid of the autonomic nervous system, controls hot and cold. The autonomic system is connected to the brain via the spinal cord, and consequently the autonomic nervous system is affected when the spinal cord is damaged.

On very hot days the increase in body temperature can be proved by taking the temperature rectally, and a rise of a degree or two is quite usual. If the temperature is taken under the tongue in these circumstances it does not always register any increase. The effect of the increase on patients is most unpleasant, similar to having a temperature caused by infection. Other effects will include: constant thirst, loss of appetite, and claustrophobia. There may also be a severe feeling of being hot and bothered, and possibly blackouts due to reduced blood pressure. This may result in a feeling of complete physical and mental exhaustion.

There is a natural tendency to reduce body temperature by drinking excessive cold fluid. This can lead to further complications. There are other more satisfactory methods to cool down. Sponge cold water over the face and body and sit or lie in front of an electric fan – this simulates normal sweating. Wear light, loose cotton clothes. Do not drink anything hot and eat only light foods such as fruit and salad. Take extra salt. Drink cold fluids regularly and try to avoid drinking vast quantities.

During excessively hot periods patients with high lesions in particular should avoid direct sunlight altogether. If it is necessary to go out, a straw hat or similar head covering should be worn for protection and a battery fan taken along for emergencies. In very hot climates most people need air conditioning, and it may be essential to patients with high lesions. This should be remembered if holidays abroad are planned.

The effect of cold is the complete reverse. Normally someone feeling cold will shiver, which is nature's way of making muscles work to produce heat. The flow of blood is redirected away from the skin's surface. Blood vessels close down to a minimum thereby conserving heat and this leaves limbs 'blue with cold'. To overcome this, able-bodied people will rub their hands together and flap their arms to increase circulation.

In a paralysed person the blood still flows at the same rate on a cold day. Consequently it is quickly cooled by the cold skin and there is rapid heat loss which leaves internal organs unprotected. If the body temperature is allowed to drop too much, the function of internal organs will be affected and patients will become seriously ill. This condition, known as hypothermia, results in death for many elderly people during unusually cold spells. Should this condition affect paraplegics, going to bed in a warm room is the most satisfactory method of regaining body heat. Remember: **no** hot water bottles or electric blankets.

Other effects of extreme cold include: the risk of frostbite, stiffness of joints and limbs, and possible low urine output. Poor concentration and a general feeling of being unwell may also result.

People who do not understand the needs of a paraplegic are often heard to say, 'Oh you will be all right on a hot or cold day because you can't feel.' This is true to a point. You will not feel hot or cold on the paralysed parts of the body. Neither will excessive heat or cold bother you too much for very short periods. But once exposed to either, for prolonged periods, the blood quickly takes up the surrounding temperature and you will feel the effects of extreme heat or cold. These effects are potentially harmful and certainly most unpleasant, so try and avoid them.

3
Pressure Sores

Regrettably there are still many who refer to pressure sores as bed sores. This is misleading and does not help in the education of their true cause. While it is possible to get sores in bed it is not the bed that causes them.

Pressure sores are caused by what their name implies, *pressure*. A simple way to demonstrate this is to apply pressure with the thumb of one hand, on the back of the other hand. Continue pressing for 30 seconds and when the thumb is removed a white mark will remain. This is where blood has been forced away from the skin by pressure and had this continued for several hours, the skin and underlying tissue would have died through being starved of its blood supply. This is the start of a pressure sore.

Exactly the same thing happens when sitting or lying in the same position for prolonged periods of time. Blood is forced away from the areas under pressure due to body weight. Because of paralysis there is no advance warning of this pressure build-up by pain or discomfort, which is nature's way of telling us to move. There is a very good example of this advance warning system in the sleep of an able-bodied person. The moment he becomes uncomfortable, a message is sent to the brain from the nerves under pressure. A reflex action takes place and the person turns over during sleep; this removes pressure and permits blood to flow freely.

Blood is our lifeline; without it we would die. If the supply is cut off from areas of our body through pressure, then that area will die. A pressure sore is exactly that; an area of tissue which has died through pressure cutting off the blood supply.

HOW TO RECOGNIZE THE START OF A PRESSURE SORE

Pressure sores do not appear instantly or without logical reason. They occur more easily in newly injured and sick patients, due to shock and poor circulation. This is why these patients are turned more frequently.

The first sign of a pressure sore is redness over the area of skin that has been in contact with the mattress or cushion. If this does not completely disappear after a few hours' relief by turning and still more pressure is applied by further lying or sitting in the same position, the skin will turn bluish-red and may even break. This might only be a small area initially and the patient may think there is nothing to worry about. If, however, still further pressure is continued, the area will turn bluish-black and will enlarge. There will be more skin loss and possibly infection. If more pressure is applied, deeper layers of underlying tissue will die; infection will penetrate deeper and throughout a wider area and if it is not treated, may enter the bone, resulting in severe and dangerous osteomyelitis.

Pressure sores can start in other ways, such as knocks and scrapes when transferring from bed to chair and from chair to car. Knocks may bruise tissue and the damage under the skin will not be noticed. If pressure is then applied through sitting or lying on such an area, a sore will develop under the skin. The reason is that such ruptured blood vessels, i.e. bruises, have not been able to heal and feed the surrounding tissue, which then dies.

Sores can start through septic spots, which are usually caused by a combination of pressure and skin bacteria that are always present. Pressure applied to a septic spot encourages the infection to spread, thus damaging a larger area. The pressure can be caused by creases in clothing, cushion covers, sheets or pillow cases. Creases in clothing can crack the skin, exposing it to bacteria. Moist skin is more easily bruised and broken, therefore it is vital not to sit or lie on wet clothing or sheets. Too much talcum powder applied after bathing is another danger. Powder can become hard and lumpy, causing pressure, so it should be used sparingly.

Another type of sore caused through pressure is known as a bursa. This is a pocket of fluid that collects between tissue and bone. It is probably caused by prolonged sitting over a period of time. This not only adds up to pressure of the normal kind, but also does not give pressure areas sufficient rest periods. Such pockets of fluid can be felt as jelly-like lumps over bony points. Sometimes the area will be red and swollen and the skin may also feel hot to touch.

Treatment of sores and bursae that have been allowed to develop is best carried out in specialized centres, for they will require skilled nursing for lengthy periods and possibly surgery.

PREVENTION OF PRESSURE SORES

It is alarming to realize that after over 30 years proven treatment of the patient with a spinal cord injury, some members of the medical profession are still under the misapprehension that pressure sores are an integral part of paralysis (Frankel, 1975). At one time this was assumed. But let me make it quite clear that it is *not* so. *Once pressure sores and their causes are fully understood, prevention is relatively simple.*

The answer to the problem lies in the name itself 'pressure sores', or sores caused by pressure. To prevent sores one has to learn to copy the able-bodied and constantly relieve pressure. 'Pressure minded' is a phrase often used to good effect. Awareness of pressure starts in the wards, where newly injured patients, regardless of the extent of injury, are turned day and night at regular intervals.

TURNING

The need for regular turning is constantly explained by nursing staff. Consequently, by the time patients are ready to sit in their wheelchairs, the need for regular lifts to prevent sores should be imprinted on their minds. Today some patients are issued with 'ripple' seat cushions and mattresses, and sheepskins, as well as normal standard sorbo-rubber wheelchair cushions. However, it should be clearly understood that these items are only aids to prevent pressure sores. There is no substitute for

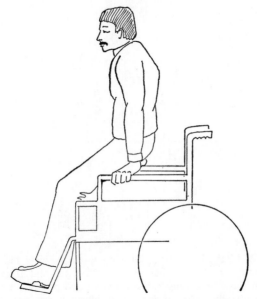

3/1. Method of lifting with complete thoracic lesion.
Patient is able to lift with normal hands and arms.

turning when in bed and for lifting when in the wheelchair. This allows blood to flow freely and feed the underlying tissue and skin. I repeat. *There is no substitute for turning in bed and lifting when in the wheelchair.*

Some patients find they can sit or lie in one position longer than others without causing damage. This is because no two people are alike. Some have more fat or padding over pressure areas than others; circulation varies from person to person and is also affected by the cord injury. Patients with limbs that are spastic often have better circulation, for the involuntary contractions of muscles help to pump blood around the system. On the other hand, these involuntary movements may cause continuous rubbing over prominent areas, thereby causing sores.

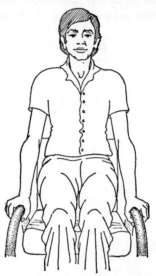

3/2. Method of lifting with complete cervical lesion below C6. Patient has no normal hand and triceps muscles. By locking hands on tyres and pressing arms against the sides of the chair, lifting is achieved by pushing down with the shoulders. Not all cervical lesions at this level can lift in the manner described, some find it necessary to transfer their weight from one buttock to the other.

Patients must learn how long they can sit or lie in one position without causing damage. This can only be done by trial and close examination of pressure areas after every turn and on return to bed. A good way of starting is by lying for 2 hours at a time when in bed, and after turning, the pressure areas should be examined with the aid of a mirror. The time between turns may be increased by 30 minutes until the maximum period is reached without any adverse effects to the skin. A maximum of 4 hours is the recommended period between turns.

In the sitting position the situation is different. The aim is to stay up in the wheelchair for a regular day. To achieve this a more frequent pattern of lifting has to be dopted. Paraplegic

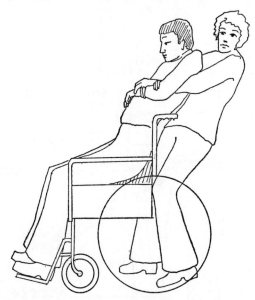

3/3. Method of lifting for complete C4 lesion. Patient has to be lifted by an attendant, for they have no arm movements. Note position of attendant's feet.

should aim at lifting themselves every 15 minutes, supporting their weight for at least 20 seconds. Remember that circulation is not at its best, so the blood takes longer to return to the area under pressure (Fig. 3/1 and 3/2).

Tetraplegics are not always able to lift themselves. Some learn to transfer their weight from side to side and this is quite satisfactory. Those unable to do this much, will require the help of an assistant to lift them (Fig. 3/3 and Plate 3/2). Tetraplegics

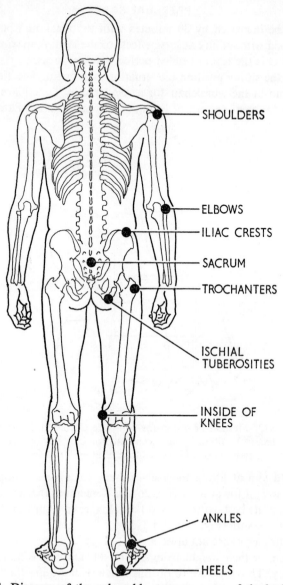

SHOULDERS

ELBOWS

ILIAC CRESTS

SACRUM

TROCHANTERS

ISCHIAL
TUBEROSITIES

INSIDE OF
KNEES

ANKLES

HEELS

3/4. Diagram of the vulnerable pressure areas of the body.

therefore have a more difficult job to find out how long they can sit without being lifted. This is best overcome by sitting for increasing periods and closely examining the skin with a mirror on return to bed. Most tetraplegic patients should be able to sit for three hourly periods without lifts and others will find the 'ripple' cushion and other aids can extend this period even further (see p. 114–7).

Many tetraplegics and some paraplegics find difficulty in examining their pressure areas because of limited movements and may require an assistant to hold a mirror. This may prove awkward and impractical, but they must not assume that an assistant will take responsibility for their skin. It is a patient's personal responsibility to check his or her own pressure areas.

It is vital to examine pressure areas on return to bed. Any redness should be noted and relieved of all pressure. Should the redness persist next day, under **no** circumstances get up. Stay in bed relieving all pressure on the area until it is completely better. The same applies if there is loss of skin or bruising. A few days spent in bed to repair minor damage, can save months in hospital later if the early danger signs are ignored.

Every part of the body is prone to pressure sores, some areas being more vulnerable than others due to the shape of our skeleton. Where sharp and protruding bones are near the skin's surface and in direct contact with a mattress or seat cushion, then these are the areas most subject to pressure sores (Fig. 3/4).

SITTING

In the sitting position, the bony points on either side of the anus, called the ischial tuberosities (which form the base of the pelvis) are the points most prone to pressure. These should be closely examined with a mirror on return to bed (Fig. 3/5).

The feet, particularly toes, backs of heels and ankles are areas most frequently damaged when sitting in a wheelchair. These areas are often damaged by careless use of footrests, and allowing legs to drop onto the footrests without looking. Feet slipping over the edges of footrests can result in the backs of heels becoming scraped, while the backs of legs and surfaces of knees and elbows are examples of other areas subject to pressure by knocks and scrapes when sitting in the wheelchair.

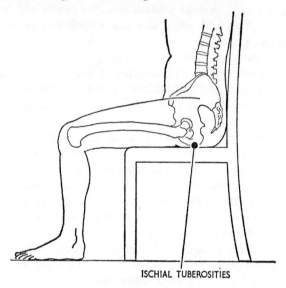

ISCHIAL TUBEROSITIES

3/5. Diagram of the vulnerable pressure areas when sitting.

Transferring from chair to bed, or in and out of cars, can result in hips becoming scraped or knocked. All these areas must be closely examined on return to bed and always before getting up the next day. Constant examination of skin and pressure areas must be strictly adhered to. The first time they are ignored can be the moment when trouble starts.

LYING

When lying in bed, pressure areas can be protected in many ways. A good quality mattress must always be used, and this should be either spring-interior or sorbo-rubber. When lying

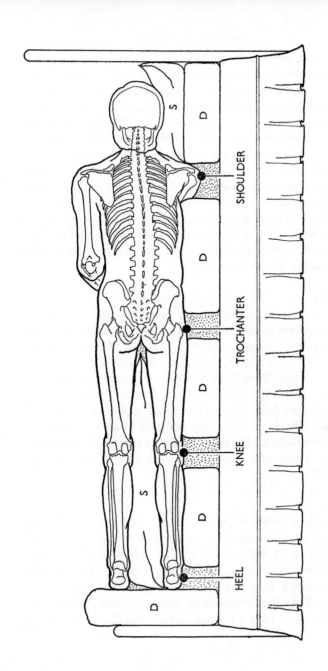

3/6. Diagram of a pack bed for use on divan or home bed.
S = single pillow.   D = double pillow in 1 case.

on the back, pillows should be placed between the knees and under the calves to suspend heels, also against the soles of the feet to prevent 'foot drop' (Fig 3/6). When lying on the side, pillows should be placed between knees and feet. If difficulties have been experienced with pressure over the hips, it will be necessary to lie on double pillows (two pillows in one pillow or bolster case) with pressure points suspended over the gaps.

Patients with scars from old sores may have difficulty in finding suitable positions in which to lie. Some may find it necessary to lie prone i.e. on their stomachs. If this position can be tolerated, it is most satisfactory and one that permits much longer periods without being turned. Care must be taken when lying prone, especially with urinals and drainage tubes, also in positioning feet and knee caps.

Pack beds

Patients undergoing treatment for pressure sores in a special centre, may have to lie on a bed constructed of 'packs' or blocks of sorbo-rubber bound together with rubber sheets. These are placed in wooden trays and positioned across the bed frame. Patients can then lie with all pressure areas suspended over the gaps (Fig. 3/7). Figs. 3/1–7 illustrate how easy it is to protect pressure points from excessive pressure, and how to avoid it altogether. There are many aids available to help patients prevent pressure sores. Like the 'ripple' seat there is also a 'ripple' mattress. These aids, and others, are fully discussed later (see p. 101).

Clothing

A very careful choice of clothing is all important in preventing pressure sores. Shoes should always be a size or two larger, made of a soft material, and not tied tightly. This allows for swelling which often occurs through lack of movement. If feet and legs continue to swell it may be necessary to wear knee-length elastic stockings. Your doctor should be consulted about this problem. Trousers should have all waist buttons and the back pockets

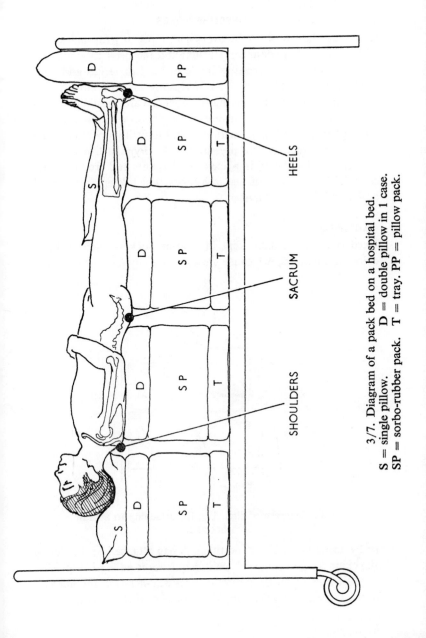

3/7. Diagram of a pack bed on a hospital bed.
S = single pillow.   D = double pillow in 1 case.
SP = sorbo-rubber pack.   T = tray.   PP = pillow pack.

removed. They must not be over-tight, especially for males who will require extra room for a urinal and the need to guard testicles from damage. Trousers made of hard materials and with thick seams should be avoided. If zips are inserted into trouser leg seams to allow the wearing of calipers, care should be taken to ensure that such zips do not cause pressure. Some types of underpants are too tight, or ride up in the sitting position, causing creases which lead to pressure marks. Pyjama trousers (not nylon) are widely used in place of underpants and are most successful. These can be tucked into socks, which keep them pulled down and free of creases.

Hard objects
Hard objects normally kept in trouser pockets such as keys, coins, and lighters, will cause pressure, even by their own weight,

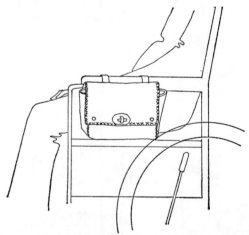

3/8. Diagram of chair bag for attaching to arm of
wheelchair.

or by accidentally sitting on them. A bag attached to the side of the chair for carrying such daily requisites is advised (Fig. 3/8).

Prevention of pressure sores is a daily 24-hour job for 365 days a year. Once a routine has been established it becomes second nature. Until then, constant thought must be given to lifting or being lifted, turning in bed and regular examination of pressure areas. Both patients and their families must clearly understand the dangers to health through pressure sores. They are potential sources of infection that can lead to loss of blood and precious protein. Infection can affect all bodily systems. Indeed, extreme cases of sores can account for the death of a patient.

HOME TREATMENT OF MINOR SORES

All paralysed people should keep a first aid kit handy to treat minor knocks and scrapes that will certainly occur from time to time. A basic kit should include the following:

a good clean container

a sharp pair of scissors

a roll of Elastoplast

packets of sterile gauze swabs

a small roll of cotton wool

a bottle of acriflavine

a bottle of Savlon, or similar antiseptic

a bottle of ether meth (to remove plaster marks, use sparingly, take care to prevent fire – highly inflammable)

a packet of Band-Aid dressings

a clinical thermometer

This is a basic kit, patients will obviously add other items as required. All the items listed can be obtained from a chemist shop. They should be readily available in the event of a knock or scrape, red mark and broken skin, or after a night out when the need for lifting was forgotten!

Do not sit or lie on the area. Go to bed and stay there until it is completely better.

METHOD   Clean the whole affected area with Savlon or a similar antiseptic; clean the surrounding skin with ether meth and if the skin is broken, cover with a dressing of sterile swabs and acriflavine, secured with Elastoplast. It is important to use a reasonable padding of swabs, ensuring that the dressing is not too tightly strapped down, for this will only add further pressure. Inspect the area after 24 hours and if necessary repeat the treatment until the sore is better. Should there be no sign of healing after 3 days, or if the dressings look dirty, the sore may be infected. Advice from your family doctor or district nurse should be obtained.

There are no hard and fast rules about which medications should or should not be used in these circumstances. Often medications used in hospital are not available from the local chemist. Most paraplegics will have obtained something that suits them. A preparation that I have found excellent is an ointment called Fucidin. Minor scrapes will usually heal without any problem once pressure is removed. If a bruise will not disappear or if it looks worse after a few days rest, treatment in hospital might be required so . . . consult your doctor.

Septic spots, sometimes caused by skin bacteria and pressure, are a common problem. In certain cases they can be quite serious, requiring continuous rest in bed. Where they persist, try washing the troubled area twice daily with pHisohex soap. This is obtainable from chemists. Should this fail, then your doctor must be consulted.

In summary:

Sores are caused through pressure.

Ensure regular turns in bed.

Check skin for damage after every turn.

Check skin for damage before getting up.

Do not sit or lie on any damaged area.

If in doubt, stay in bed with weight off the suspect area.

Ensure regular lifts in the wheelchair.

Do not depend on any mechanical aid to prevent pressure.

Do not wear over-tight clothing.

Avoid sitting or lying on a wet cushion or bed.

Keep well away from open fires or hot pipes.

Check your skin for damage on return to bed.

Reference
Frankel, H.L. (1975). Traumatic Paraplegia, *Nursing Mirror*, 6 November.

4

Bowel Management

Management of the bowels is undoubtedly the most distressing aspect of paraplegia, especially to the newly injured. The aim is to regulate bowel action to occur regularly at the same time, either daily, or on alternate days. This is vitally important in good rehabilitation for obvious social and domestic reasons. Although most paraplegics are incontinent, bowel action can be controlled and regulated with a combination of sensible eating and drinking, aperients, suppositories, automatic reflex bowel action or manual evacuation.

The secret of good bowel management lies in regular, sensible eating and drinking habits. It is impossible to say exactly what people should or should not eat or drink, for no two people are exactly the same. For example, if by eating curry the bowels are upset, or by eating eggs they become constipated, then these foods should obviously be avoided.

Most people prefer to attend to their bowels on alternate days. This seems the most satisfactory routine. By taking an aperient the night before, faeces are moved into the lower bowel and the rectum ready for emptying. The upper bowel will then be empty and the risk of accidents and constipation reduced.

There are many different types of aperients available and some suit one person, but not others. There are no hard and fast rules governing the type to take. As long as a good result and a formed stool is obtained without accidents in between, then the individual choice is satisfactory. Difficulty may arise in measuring the exact dosage, too much can upset the bowels, whilst too little can produce a small result and possible constipation.

Senokot tablets are widely used in paraplegia and are very successful, and the dosage can be easily measured to suit individual needs. Other aperients in common use include Senokot granules, syrup of figs, Dulcolax and cascara. Having taken an appropriate aperient the previous evening, suppositories are given before emptying the bowel. These are of two main types, Dulcolax and glycerine. Both are designed to aid the rectum to empty by stimulating it to contract automatically. Dulcolax suppositories promote a stronger action but take longer to act; up to one and a half hours compared with 30 minutes for the glycerine. Some patients may experience slight side effects from the use of suppositories, these may include stomach cramps and temporary rise in blood pressure with a slight headache (autonomic dysreflexia). Such effects usually only last during the time the bowel is contracting to empty.

Those patients who have developed fully automatic bowel actions, usually with the aid of Dulcolax suppositories, will avoid the need for manual evacuation. This is always more satisfactory and certainly causes less inconvenience. Others usually require manual evacuation of the bowel with the aid of glycerine suppositories. These are inserted into the rectum 30 minutes before the actual evacuation. Great care should be taken when doing this; a little petroleum jelly aids insertion, which should be upwards and towards the umbilicus, which is the natural position of the anal canal.

Manual evacuation whether carried out by the patient or by an attendant, must be done very gently using one gloved finger only. Nails should be kept short, to prevent damage to the lining of the rectum. If the evacuation is being carried out with the patient lying on the bed, he should be placed on the left side with the buttocks at 90 degrees to the mattress. A plastic sheet and cellulose wadding should be placed under the buttocks, ensuring that bedclothes are well protected. Holding the patient steady with the left hand, one well lubricated gloved finger of the right hand should gently be eased into the rectum, rotated and withdrawn, bringing the faeces out with it. Between each insertion a few seconds should elapse, allowing the bowel to contract on its own, which then brings the faeces down closer to the anus. This procedure should be continued until all traces of faeces have been removed. Clean cellulose wadding should be placed under the buttocks and the patient left for a while to ensure that the motion has finished. Moist cotton wool is recommended to clean the buttocks after evacuation, paper being too hard and more difficult to handle.

Obviously this procedure is not pleasant for the attendant, and is equally embarrassing for the patient. Attendants should wear protective clothing: a plastic apron, suitable plastic or rubber gloves and a paper face mask if required. A window should be opened and a fresh air spray used afterwards.

Under normal circumstances the alternative of giving enemas (the washing out of the bowels) is not recommended in paraplegia. Due to sensation loss and possible weakness of the bowel wall, damage can result.

Paraplegics and low level tetraplegics should be able to transfer on and off the lavatory, where they can attend to their own bowels, and when this is possible, it is obviously the most satisfactory method. Under these circumstances aperients and suppositories will still be required, but there is one advantage in this position and that is gravity. Excessive straining and sitting for prolonged periods should be avoided, for this can cause haemorrhoids and possible prolapse of the rectum. Both conditions are not uncommon in paraplegia, and in the event of rectal bleeding consult your doctor.

Various aids to bowel management can be obtained on prescription. These include: a suitable aperient, Dulcolax or glycerine suppositories, disposable rubber or plastic gloves, plastic sheets, cellulose wadding, and hospital quality cotton wool.

Other aids include inflatable toilet seats which ought to be used (Plate 4/1), commode chairs, hoists and handrails. These can be obtained through the local Department of Social Services in the patient's home area.

For tetraplegics, who have limited hand movements, there is a suppository applicator and full details can be obtained from the Occupational Therapy Department, Rehabilitation Education Center, Oak Street, At Stadium Drive, Champaign, Illinois 61820, U.S.A. The Disabled Living Foundation has complete toilet layouts, including a combined toilet and bidet. Visits can be arranged by appointment to try the equipment. It should be noted that if patients wish to use a bidet, great care must be taken to ensure only warm water is used, thus preventing burns!

Problems often arise in disposing of soiled materials, and it is unwise to try and flush everything down the lavatory for fear of blockage. Most local authorities have a 'Green Bag' service, where soiled materials can be collected in the bag provided. The social services department should be able to supply full details. Many patients choose to purchase an incinerator and burn soiled materials, and where this is possible, it is perhaps the best solution.

CONSTIPATION

Constipation is a common complaint amongst paraplegics. It may be the cause of headaches, sweating and sometimes a slight rise in temperature, and if persistent, constipation can lead to other complications such as bladder dysfunction and infection of the urinary system.

Short bouts of constipation are usually caused by changes of diet, daily routine, poor fluid intake or certain drugs such as codeine and some antibiotics. Quick relief can be obtained by taking extra measures of the chosen aperient and having the bowels evacuated daily until a normal pattern is re-established. Invariably patients with automatic bowels will require manual evacuation should they become constipated. Many patients make the mistake after being discharged from hospital of allowing themselves to become constipated, thinking this will prevent possible accidents. On the contrary, constipation is often the cause of diarrhoea.

A high roughage diet in the form of fruit, vegetables, sweetcorn, tomatoes, and cereals is essential in the prevention of constipation. If relief cannot be obtained, a faecal softener or bulk former, such as Dioctal and Normacol, may be required. These are available on prescription, and the family doctor should be consulted.

5

Management of the Urinary System

The urinary system consists of two kidneys, left and right, connected to the bladder by tubes called ureters. The bladder empties through the urethra, which lies through the centre of the penis in males (see Fig. 5/1). Urine is the waste fluid secreted by the kidneys, and passes down the ureters into the bladder, where it is stored until ready for excreting via the urethra (this is the act of micturition). The production and secretion of urine by the kidneys is a process designed to filter impurities from the blood. It is therefore necessary to drink adequate amounts of fluid to keep the blood free of impurities and the urinary system flushed, especially when paralysed.

The urinary system is a delicate, sensitive part of the body and in a paralysed person is more prone to complications. To prevent unnecessary complications great care must be constantly observed and a full understanding of its function learned. Recognizing symptoms of problems, and knowing what action to take is essential to survival.

The bladder acts as a reservoir for urine. When it is full, urine is expelled by the muscular action of its component called the detrusor. Its opening is controlled by two sphincters (circular muscles at the bladder neck), one internal the other external. As the detrusor muscle contracts to empty a full bladder, the internal sphincter opens allowing the urine to pass. Able-bodied people can feel the distension of the bladder before micturition: they also have control of the external sphincter to check the out-flow

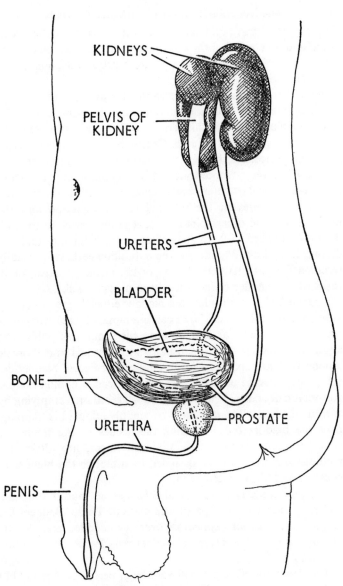

KIDNEYS

PELVIS OF
KIDNEY

URETERS

BLADDER

BONE

URETHRA

PENIS

PROSTATE

5/1. urinary system in the male.

if necessary. When paralysed, there is no normal warning sensation and no control of the external sphincter (other than in the case of some incomplete lesions), and a urine collection device has to be used.

Immediately following injury to the spinal cord, the bladder emptying mechanism is nonfunctional due to spinal shock. To empty the bladder during this period a catheter will be passed, and at the National Spinal Injuries Centre, Stoke Mandeville Hospital, this procedure, known as 'intermittent catheterisation' is carried out three or more times daily in conjunction with regulated drinking. Particular care is taken to do this under sterile conditions to prevent the introduction of infection into the bladder. In some other spinal units, it is the policy to treat all the newly injured with an indwelling catheter giving continual drainage. At Stoke Mandeville the indwelling catheter is usually reserved for patients with defects of the urinary system, or in cases where bladder training has been unsuccessful.

As spinal shock subsides, the bladder either begins to empty automatically (like a baby's) or can be emptied by applying pressure over the lower abdomen above the symphysis pubis. The automatic bladder develops usually with cervical and thoracic lesions that are spastic. An autonomous or flaccid bladder develops with flaccid paralysis, usually with cauda equina lesions. Automatic or spastic bladders can be triggered into emptying by various methods. The one most commonly adopted is 'tapping' over the bladder area; stroking the insides of the thighs, or stimulating the rectum with a gloved finger, are alternative methods. All methods are designed to stimulate the bladder to contract and allow micturition.

The autonomous or flaccid bladder has no muscle tone and will not react to this type of stimulation. These bladders are emptied by manual expression over the bladder area, or by abdominal straining, since abdominal muscles usually function in these lesions.

The degree of efficiency will vary from person to person, but once a satisfactory method is found, patients are trained to empty their bladders every 3 hours. The objects are the establishment of a good system of emptying the bladder and the reduction of residual urine to below 100ml. The prevention of infection and other complications of a high residual urine, and the ability to prevent incontinence interfering with rehabilitation and social activities are important.

URINALS

The male paraplegic should regard himself as fortunate in having a penis onto which it is possible to attach a urinal, which can be one of several different types. This is often taken for granted and the need for regular expression of the bladder forgotten. Over the years this can lead to a lazy and weak bladder that becomes difficult to manage. It is therefore important to stress that the bladder, whether of the automatic or autonomous type, should be expressed every 2 to 3 hours, or even hourly if the patient drinks plenty of fluids.

The majority of men will choose to wear the condom type urinal attached to a G.U. suprapubic bag which is commonly called a 'kipper'. There are other suitable urinals for the male paraplegic such as the Stoke Mandeville Hospital Type and the Thackery Male Urinal. The Stoke Mandeville type, made by Down Bros, Mayer & Phelps Ltd., Church Path, Mitcham, Surrey, CR4 3VE, has a detachable penile sheath supplied in various sizes from approximately 22mm (7/8in) to 38mm (1½in). The sheath is first applied to the penis, without any skin adhesive, then attached to the urinal which is fixed to the waist and leg by straps. This urinal, although suitable for many, has its drawbacks. The sheath sometimes causes pressure to the penis. It can also easily become detached when transferring to and from a wheelchair or in the event of the penis becoming erect. The Thackery urinal is very similar in construction, fitting and in the drawbacks.

The condom type urinal is different from the others in that the sheath is fixed to the penis by skin adhesive. This reduces the risk of it becoming detached and would certainly seem the most satisfactory. Condoms should be changed at least every 24 hours as instructed.

A small number of people may find that they are allergic to either the skin adhesive or the rubber sheath. This might occur after several years' use. Should this happen, a special nylon sheath is available together with a non-allergic adhesive called Dow Corning Medical Adhesive B; this is produced in the U.S.A. and is available in the U.K. An alternative non-allergic adhesive is Saltair Ostomy adhesive solution, produced by Salt & Son Ltd., 220 Corporation Street, Birmingham, 4. Further research is being conducted into finding more suitable adhesives and condom sheaths. In the meantime the nylon sheath and both adhesives are available on prescription.

Prolonged erections can cause pressure sores from the rubber ring of the condom. To prevent this, after the condom has been fitted cut the ring with a pair of scissors. When fitting a condom, always ensure that at least 2·5cm (1in) of free condom is left to prevent pressure on the end of the penis from the plastic button.

It is of prime importance that both tubing and plastic buttons are sterilized before fitting. In the home this can be done either by boiling for 5 minutes, or by soaking overnight in 16% Dakin's solution or a weak solution of household bleach. Before sterilizing tubes and buttons, they should be thoroughly cleaned in hot soapy water. Mineral deposits on plastic buttons can be removed by soaking in 5% hydrochloric acid. Condoms are disposable.

Application of condom urinal

To apply a condom urinal the equipment required is: a condom sheath, condom rubber tubing approximately 12·5cm (5in) long, a plastic condom connecting button, an orange stick or 'pricker', gauze swabs, or cotton wool, ether meth, skin adhesive, and the urinal or 'kipper'.

METHOD   Gently remove the old condom taking care not to damage the skin; if it is difficult to remove, use ether meth to dissolve the adhesive. Thoroughly clean all traces of adhesive from the penis with a swab and ether meth, then wash the penis and scrotal area with warm soapy water. Dry carefully and examine the penis for skin damage. Should there be skin damage, a fresh condom must **not** be affixed. Cover the damaged area with a sterile dressing and stay in bed using a glass or disposable urine bottle until the skin is completely healed.

The new condom and tubing should be assembled ready for application. This is achieved by placing the plastic button in the end of the condom, then pushing it into the rubber tubing. The rubber of the condom which then lies across the end of the plastic button is pricked out leaving the way clear for the free flow of urine. A moderate coat of adhesive should then be applied to the shaft of the penis, waiting a few seconds for it to become tacky before rolling the condom down the shaft of the penis. Whilst doing this a little pressure from the fingers will aid adhesion. The best results are obtained if the condom is fitted to an erect penis.

In some spinal units patients are instructed to attach the condom to the base of the penis using Elastoplast rather than skin adhesive. The disadvantage of this practice is the possibility of the condom becoming detached and the danger of skin damage when removing the Elastoplast.

After the sheath is fitted, the rubber tubing can be attached either to a bag worn on the leg for sitting in the wheelchair, or to a disposable drainage bag hung on the side of the bed.

There are several different types of urine collection bags on the market. The Bardic 'Dispoz-a-bag' is plastic and disposable, and can be worn either on the leg or fixed to the bed. The other bag in regular use is the G.U. suprapubic bag, or 'kipper', which can be used daily and washed ready for the next day.

Condoms, adhesive (Warne adhesive), plastic connector buttons and rubber tubing are supplied by the Department of Health and Social Security, Government Buildings, Warbreck

Hill Road, Blackpool, Lancashire. Patients are given a certificate on their discharge from hospital stating that they wear a condom urinal. This should be sent to the Department of Health with the initial request for supplies. Disposable and G.U. suprapubic bags are obtainable on prescription from the family doctor.

URINARY PROBLEMS FACING WOMEN

So far, no-one has been able to invent a suitable urinal for the female paraplegic. Some have been produced, but all cause pressure and should be avoided. Consequently females have to work very hard indeed to develop a good automatic or autonomous bladder, together with very strict drinking and bladder emptying routines.

Women faced with this problem usually succeed better than men in organizing their bladder routine, for obvious social reasons. Those physically able to use the lavatory, do so every 3 hours, expressing the bladder in the normal way. Others may use a female urine receiver sitting in the chair, or may lie on the bed. To prevent possible accidents in between times, females wear absorbent pads and plastic pants. These are available through the social services, and you should contact your social worker or district nurse for full details. More attractive pants than those supplied on the National Health Service can be bought from firms such as Basingstoke Hygiene Products (U.K.) Ltd., 2b, Amity Road, Reading, Berkshire, and women may wish to consider buying these themselves.

Problems obviously arise when taking part in social activities such as shopping, going to the theatre, eating in restaurants, in finding suitable places to express the bladder. Special consideration is necessary when travelling. At such times many females choose not to drink at all. This certainly may prevent them getting wet, but often leads to infection of the bladder and further problems. It is better to decrease the amount of drinking before going out, then compensate for it later by drinking extra fluid on return home. A little research and a few telephone calls are easily made to find out if a particular place has either accessible toilets, or a satisfactory room that can be used. Do not wait until you arrive, to find there is nothing suitable. This can only lead to bad temper, frustration, getting wet and the risk of pressure sores.

SUPRAPUBIC BAG REF GU 532 'THE KIPPER'

The kipper urinal cannot be sterilized; it can only be disinfected and therefore it is necessary to have two – one on and one off. The kipper can be used with the condom urinal, and by men and women who require an indwelling catheter.

After use, the screw top should be removed and the urinal drained and rinsed in warm water. The urinal should be thoroughly washed in warm soapy water, rinsed and left to soak for 2 to 3 hours in a 16% Dakin's solution. If this is not available, a 5% solution of household bleach can be used and in which case the urinal should not be soaked for more than 2 hours.

Careful attention should be paid in cleaning the screw top and the drain tap. Where mineral deposits are found, a fine brush may be required to clean the holes. After soaking, urinals should again be rinsed in warm water and finally hung up to dry with the drainage tap open.

Urinals should not be exposed to direct heat or the rubber will perish. Normally they will last 6 months with careful use. The rubber first starts to perish near the tap, so regular inspection is advised.

Patients are well advised always to carry a spare urinal plus condom whenever they are away from their home, no matter how short the journey.

DRINKING

Unless instructed otherwise, patients should aim at maintaining a high non-alcoholic fluid intake of 3 litres (5 pints) or more in 24 hours. This is all important when paralysed as it prevents stagnation of urine which leads to infection. A concentrated urine will deposit minerals in the system, leading to the formation of stones, and together with bad emptying of the bladder encourages infection.

Alcohol, especially spirits, and spices are bad for the kidneys and should not be taken, for the following reasons. Firstly, due to paralysis the circulation is reduced and this includes circulation through the kidneys. Making the kidneys work harder by drinking alcohol and eating spices such as pepper, curry and some sauces only adds to the strain they are already under from poor circulation. Secondly, alcohol not only puts added strain on the kidneys, it has an even worse effect on bladder function. Not so many years ago alcohol was given in large quantities before crude surgery was performed, in place of an anaesthetic. Most people will have experienced the effect of too much alcohol. They become drunk, weak, lose balance and are unable to stand up properly. This is because alcohol in large quantities is a depressant poison. It also depresses the action of the automatic bladder.

Those with an automatic bladder depend on good muscle tone for its emptying. Because it works automatically, there is no normal warning sensation to indicate when it needs emptying and this cannot be helped by straining with the abdominal muscles, as with the autonomous bladder. Consequently the bladder will not empty, it overfills and becomes stretched out of shape, there is stagnation of urine which becomes infected and there is also the possible risk of kidney damage due to a build up of back pressure.

Alcohol in moderation is acceptable so are spices. A glass of beer or wine will do little harm. Spirits such as whisky, gin and brandy have a high alcohol content and should *not* be taken. Excessive alcohol also encourages forgetfulness, especially the need to lift in the chair and to empty urinals which can burst. It can cause loss of balance leading to falls from the wheelchair which may result in bone fractures.

COMPLICATIONS OF THE URINARY SYSTEM

It is of paramount importance to acquire some knowledge and understanding of the more obvious complications of the urinary system, in order to recognize possible problem symptoms and to know what action to take. It is not necessary to learn every detail about possible complications. These are numerous and best left to the medical profession to worry about. The majority of problems will be connected with infection in the following: the bladder (cystitis), the kidneys (nephritis), the pelvis of kidneys and ureters (pyelitis), and the urethra (urethritis). Other problems may include bladder retention, high residual urine, reflux of urine, and the formation of bladder and kidney stones.

BLADDER INFECTIONS

Infection in the bladder is the most common problem, and if untreated, infection of the remainder of the system can follow. Symptoms are easy to recognize, being: dirty, cloudy urine which may be foul smelling; possible bleeding from the bladder (haematuria); headache; sweating; and sickness. There may be a rise in body temperature; possible rise in pulse rate; and frequent passing of small amounts of urine with automatic bladders. Also possible is an increase in spasms; a burning sensation in the bladder (where there is sensation); and there may also be shivering and rigors but these more often occur with further infection of the urinary system.

At the first sign of infection a urine specimen collected in a sterile manner, should be sent to a hospital pathology laboratory for examination. Arrangements for this should be made with the family doctor or district nurse. To prevent infection spreading to the remainder of the system, and possibly causing a 'flare up' the family doctor may prescribe a course of antibiotics that can be changed if necessary when laboratory results are known. A flare up is the term used to describe a sudden rise in temperature, rigors and vomiting, due to infection of the urinary system. It is usually associated with pyelitis.

The urine of a paraplegic tends to be alkaline in reaction, especially if there is infection. Consequently the doctor may follow the course of antibiotics with an acidifying and antiseptic drug like ascorbic acid, or G500 (which is a mixture of methionine 250mg and hexamine mandelate 250mg), in an attempt to make the urine acid to discourage infection and stone formation.

INFECTION OF KIDNEY, PELVIS AND URETERS

One cause of infection in kidneys and ureters is infection of the bladder that has travelled back up the ureters. Other less common virulent infections may find their way to the kidneys through the circulation. Additional symptoms to bladder infections are: high rise in body temperature; high rise in pulse rate; possible rise in respiration rate; rigors, shivering and hot and cold spells; and pains in sides, back and shoulders. A definite feeling of illness will be experienced, which will mean confinement to bed for at least 24 hours after body temperature has returned to normal. As in the case of a bladder infection the family doctor should be called and a urine specimen taken.

If, as is often experienced, body temperature is very high, 2 aspirin tablets taken every 6 hours will help reduce it (soluble aspirin is more easily digested). Tetraplegics in particular will suffer, and an electric fan, sponging and cold drinks will all help to reduce body temperature. The added risk of pressure sores *must* be remembered at such times, hence the need for more frequent turns.

Kidney infections are dangerous and should not be ignored, for if they are not treated immediately permanent damage will result impairing their function. Repeated infections of either kidneys or bladder require investigation, since causes can usually be treated if discovered in time. The need for regular check-ups to monitor kidney function is essential (see p. 89).

KIDNEY AND BLADDER STONES

The formation of stones in either the bladder or the kidneys is not uncommon in paraplegia and is usually associated with infection, the use of indwelling catheters, or low fluid intake.

During the early months following injury there is a higher risk of stone formation. This is because calcium is given off from the bones due to lack of movement and weight-bearing. This is then excreted by the kidneys in the urine. With a combination of infection, low fluid intake and output, together with excess calcium there is a chance of deposits being formed in the urinary system, leading to the growth of stones. This can be reduced to a minimum by regular drinking, turning, and careful catheterisation to prevent infection. Milk is rich in calcium and should be restricted at all times, especially during the early months following injury.

The formation of stones can be clearly seen on X-ray when having an intravenous pyelogram (I.V.P.). Should they be discovered, their removal will be determined by the spinal specialist. It is less likely for stones to form in a sterile acid urine, which again emphasizes the need for the system to be kept free of infection.

People who require permanent indwelling catheters usually have chronic bladder infection and become more prone to stone formations. This is because mineral crystals in the urine tend to collect on the balloon of the catheter. These then grow together forming a stone. To reduce this risk daily bladder washouts must be given and catheters changed as instructed (see p. 70).

INFECTION OF URETHRA

Infection of the urethra can occur without infection to the remainder of the urinary system, although it is usually associated with at least an infection of the bladder. Those requiring permanent indwelling catheters are most prone to this condition, because the infection is introduced during catheter changes.

Symptoms of infection in the urethra are usually discharge of pus from the urethra, or from around the catheter. The condition is fairly common, especially in those having indwelling catheters. It should not be ignored because further complications can arise. In males, particularly, a fistula can form. This is a hole through the wall of the urethra caused by a combination of the infection and pressure from the catheter. The general practitioner should be consulted, and he may prescribe treatment or refer patients to a spinal specialist.

REFLUX OF URINE

Reflux of urine is simply the flowing back of urine up the ureters. When this happens, and it is usually first suspected on I.V.P. examination, the pelvis and possibly the ureter of the kidney involved become enlarged, and the patient is said to have hydro-nephrosis.

Confirmation of reflux is obtained by a special X-ray examin-ation called a cystogram. For this, the bladder is filled with a special dye through a catheter and the movement and flow of the dye can be observed with X-ray apparatus. Where a reflux has been confirmed, treatment will be determined by the spinal specialist after tests. Prevention of reflux can be helped by main-taining the urine in a sterile condition and ensuring residual is low. Regular expression of the bladder will aid this.

RESIDUAL URINE

Residual urine refers to the quantity of urine left in the bladder after it has been emptied in the normal manner. To measure this amount, a catheter is inserted into the bladder immediately after micturition, the remaining urine then being drained and carefully measured. Ideally residual urine should be less than 100ml. If it is higher, there is a possibility of infection due to stagnation, and bladder and kidney damage. Causes of high residual urine vary, the most common being obstruction in the outlet of the bladder which impedes emptying, weak muscle tone of the bladder, and failure on behalf of patients to express their bladders at regular intervals, which leads to over-stretched and weak bladders.

After full investigation of kidney and bladder function by I.V.P. and cystogram, the treatment of high residual urine will be determined by a spinal specialist. For males this might include cystoscopy (examination of bladder interior), transurethral resection (T.U.R.) – this is the removal of obstruction in the bladder neck, to widen the outlet – or dilatation of the urethra or division of the external sphincter.

Due to differences in the female anatomy, removal of a section of sphincter is not normally carried out because of technical difficulties. Where residual urine is high in females, the sphincters are usually dilated or stretched, which then allows a free flow of urine. In certain circumstances bladder function can be helped with specific drugs, as well as with very frequent and regular expression.

BLADDER RETENTION

This is quite common in paraplegia, and means that for some reason the patient is unable to empty the bladder. The causes vary, and the symptoms will include a thumping headache, sweating, increase in spasms, or the complete reverse, distended bladder, flushing of face, and possibly a slow pulse rate.

If the bladder refuses to empty by stimulation or by expression normally carried out, a doctor should be called or the patient taken to a hospital without delay. This is particularly important in patients with high thoracic and cervical lesions where, due to the over-filled bladder, there will be a reflex action on blood pressure which rises sharply and causes a thumping headache (autonomic dysreflexia). Relief for this situation will be determined by the doctor. Usually a straightforward catheterisation will be carried out to empty the bladder.

Bladder retention is often the result of travelling in a car on long journeys and particularly after drinking beer! To reduce this potential risk, limit drinking when travelling and a stretch across the seats every 2 hours will stimulate the bladder to empty. It might be worthwhile mentioning that patients considering the purchase of a motor vehicle, should seriously consider the aspect of bladder function. It is a fact that some patients do experience difficulties in emptying their bladders when sitting in certain types of motor vehicles.

Taking a urine specimen

Under ideal circumstances a urine specimen should be taken by a doctor, nurse or trained orderly. In the home this is not always possible and as it is often necessary for the paraplegic to have a urine test, I feel this aspect should be covered.

A urine specimen can be collected in two different ways; either by passing a catheter, or by collecting a mid-stream sample of urine. I will deal with the latter method first.

A MID-STREAM SAMPLE (M.S.U.)   This is taken whilst actually passing urine not when starting, and ensures that any contaminant is washed away and not collected in the jar. Particular care must be taken in preventing the jar coming in contact with skin or clothing, for this could lead to the sample becoming contaminated and thus an inaccurate laboratory result.

The equipment required for taking an M.S.U. includes a sterile urine collection jar, sterile gauze swabs, Savlon, and a kidney dish or receiver.

Approximately 45 minutes before taking the specimen, a good drink of water should be taken. The procedure should then be as follows. Thoroughly wash hands, soak a swab in Savlon, then thoroughly wash the end of the penis. This should be repeated at least three times, using a clean swab each time. The same procedure should be applied with females. Thoroughly wash the urethral area by holding the labia apart with a sterile swab. Swabbing should be from the outside and from the top in a downward direction only, working towards the urethra. Swabbing should be done at least five times, using a clean swab each time. Ensure the top of the specimen jar is not too tightly closed. Stimulate the bladder in the normal manner, and when urine is flowing freely, remove the top of the jar and insert into stream, collecting about 2·5–5cm (1–2in) of urine. Replace the lid on the jar quickly and take it to a hospital pathology laboratory as soon as possible.

Patients with indwelling catheters can obtain a specimen by clipping off the catheter for 10 to 15 minutes after a drink of water. Thoroughly wash the end of the catheter in Savlon; remove the clip and again collect a mid-stream of urine, not the first flow from the catheter.

The indwelling catheter

For various reasons, such as chronic infection, defects in the urinary system, or where the bladder is unable to expel urine and all measures to make it function have failed, drainage may become necessary by employing an indwelling catheter. There are various types that can be used. The one found to be most satisfactory at the National Spinal Injuries Centre is the Foley catheter. This is introduced through the urethra and retained in the bladder by an inflatable balloon.

To minimize infection and the formation of stones, catheters are changed twice weekly and daily bladder washouts given. Regular catheter changes also relieve pressure to the urethra, thereby reducing the risk of pressure sores. Catheterisations are normally carried out by a doctor or trained nurse. Some paraplegics living outside the hospital situation are taught to change their own catheters, and to do their own bladder washouts. As catheters sometimes block and difficulty may arise in obtaining a doctor or nurse, especially at night or weekends, those able to manage these procedures, should be encouraged.

Patients requiring indwelling catheters, will be supplied with all equipment necessary for both changing the catheter and doing daily bladder washouts. Those able to change their own catheter will receive professional advice and instruction on the technique. Others will be advised to depend on either their family doctor or district nurse, so it is unnecessary to elaborate further.

Bladder washouts can be carried out by most patients or their relatives. Understanding this technique can obviate long waits for district nurses. It may also be of value in relieving catheter blockages that often occur.

Bladder washout

Bladder washouts must be carried out under sterile conditions to prevent the introduction of infection. All equipment must be sterilized. In hospital this is usually done by a central sterilizing department which prepares all equipment needed in a pack which is hen sterilized in a large oven type receptacle called an autoclave. The user has only to open the pack and will find everything ready. At home, patients may have to resort to the old-fashioned but effective method of boiling for 5 minutes.

Daily washouts with a sterile 4% boric lotion solution keep the bladder clear of sediment and help prevent stone formation. These start as mineral crystals that grow on the catheter balloon.

Washouts are best carried out first thing in the morning. After a night's rest sediment will have collected in the bladder. Again I stress, this is a sterile procedure even if the bladder is already infected.

Equipment required will be supplied from hospital prior to discharge and will include: Stylex syringe and plastic measuring jug, receiver or kidney dish, artery forceps and gallipots, disposable gloves and face mask, sterile disposable syringes, and sterile 4% boric lotion. Large sterilizing saucepans and forceps are supplied to boil necessary equipment and these should be kept as clean as possible.

METHOD   Wearing a face mask, thoroughly scrub hands and put on sterile disposable gloves. All equipment necessary should have been previously sterilized and placed on a clean surface, such as a table or trolley swabbed with Savlon.

1. Lie catheter in receiver and swab the connection to drainage bag before parting the two.
2. Fill Stylex syringe with 60ml of warm 4% boric lotion. Expel air and inject fluid quickly into the bladder.
3. Immediately withdraw fluid to 45ml, then slowly for remaining 15ml and discard.
4. Repeat this procedure at least three times until a clear return of fluid is obtained.
5. Reconnect the catheter to the drainage bag.

If your doctor has prescribed a local antibiotic for the bladder this should be injected into the bladder through the catheter after the washout is complete, and then clipped off for 10–15 minutes with artery forceps before reconnection to the drainage bag. Usually the amount of antibiotic to be injected into the bladder will be determined by the doctor, but where no instructions are given 10–15ml is normal.

Points to note
Because of the dangers of possible reflux, it is important that only 60ml is injected into the bladder at a time.

Where there is a known reflux, 30–40ml of fluid should be injected slowly.

If a catheter is found to be blocked on washout, it should be changed without delay. Similar symptoms to retention of the bladder may well be experienced. Sometimes the balloon of a catheter fails to deflate; if the catheter is not blocked, then inject 10ml of liquid paraffin into the balloon. This should then perish during the next 12 to 24 hours, allowing the catheter to be removed in the normal manner.

Should the catheter be blocked and if it cannot be removed, patients should seek medical assistance without delay.

6
Sex

Interruption of normal sexual functions in both male and female paraplegics, has long been recognized as a serious aspect of rehabilitation. This is even more pronounced in young people who often feel inadequate. It is a normal and understandable reaction, for sexual potential is vital to everyone.

Not so many years ago, a person seen sitting in a wheelchair was assumed to be impotent. Through education and publicity this attitude is at long last changing. There are however still many members of the medical and nursing professions, the church, the general public and even patients themselves, who are shy and embarrassed to talk freely about the subject. This can only hinder complete rehabilitation.

In the majority of spinal cord injuries, an ability to experience orgasm is lost. There may also be physical, mental and social problems that inhibit relationships. Often a new approach to the whole subject is required. Sexual relations either in or out of marriage are based on more than the physical enjoyment of orgasm, although this experience is undoubtedly the fulfilment and climax of the sexual act. When this sensation has been removed an alternative outlet has to be found. A true understanding of these difficulties and how to overcome them when one partner is paralysed, no matter how seriously, is essential in finding an outlet and in maintaining a happy and contented sexual relationship. To achieve this, couples have to learn to avoid shyness and hesitancy. The paraplegic should encourage the able-bodied partner to treat him or her as a person with normal feelings of desire and love.

THE MALE

The male paraplegic is faced with two main problems; the inability to maintain an erection, and the inability to ejaculate semen containing sperms. The functions of the sexual organs are very complex, and it is impossible to group all male paraplegics together and describe just one situation. Where the spinal cord has been damaged and to what extent, will determine the sexual potential.

The nerves that supply sexual functions, stem from the lower segments of the spinal cord and therefore most patients with cord injuries will have affected sexual functions. Patients with damage to the upper segments of the cord, in particular cervical injuries, are often able to have good and lasting erections without being able to ejaculate; those with lower levels of injury may not be able to maintain an erection or produce sperms. Only patients with incomplete lesions will stand a chance of experiencing orgasm.

There is no known treatment to relieve loss of orgasm. Some patients claim to reach orgasm through stimulation of the nipple area or other parts of the body above the level of injury. Others have experienced a type of para-orgasm, or 'phantom' orgasm, but I believe this to be psychological, with the mind playing tricks recalling previous experiences.

A weak erection can sometimes be helped by the simple application of a moderately tight rubber band around the base of the penis. This often maintains the erection long enough for intercourse. This must be removed directly intercourse is finished, for fear of skin damage. If this fails, erections can sometimes be helped by drug therapy.

Males wishing to have a family, but unable to produce the necessary sperms for fertilization, should discuss the situation with a spinal specialist who will, if possible, allow the use of electrotherapy. Sometimes this will stimulate the prostate gland and produce an ejaculation. If the resultant semen is found to be suitable it can be used to impregnate the partner by artificial insemination (see p. 149). It should be made clear that only a limited number of patients will be able to produce sperm in this manner. The concentration of sperms produced will drop after several months of becoming paralysed. In the future it may be possible to collect sperm from the newly injured and these will then be kept in deep-freeze storage until children are wanted and artificial insemination is carried out.

To relieve a degree of embarrassment it should be pointed out that the majority of paraplegics who are able to have erections, do so because of a reflex action not controlled by sexual desire or will. Lack of this understanding often leads to awkward moments when paraplegics are being washed or dressed. A reflex erection is more easily obtained when the bladder is full. This might be useful to know but it is unwise to attempt intercourse with a full bladder. At such times there is a real danger of bladder retention and it might be necessary for a catheter to be passed. To avoid this, always ensure that the bladder is empty before intercourse and do not drink for an hour or two beforehand.

Males requiring indwelling catheters are advised to remove the catheter before intercourse, though some patients claim that the catheter helps to maintain an erection and this might well be true. To leave a catheter in is dangerous, for movement may pull the balloon through the sphincter of the bladder thereby causing serious damage.

Males totally unable to obtain an erection will obviously be unable to partake in intercourse of the normal kind. A technique of 'stuffing' the limp penis into the female vagina and rhythmically rubbing against the female clitoris may be sufficient to satisfy the female partner. Another alternative is to use one of the many sexual aids available (see p. 77).

THE FEMALE

The female paraplegic will usually experience a temporary upset of the menstrual cycle following injury, but this normally rectifies itself within a short period of time.

Under normal circumstances, women with either complete or incomplete lesions are able to become pregnant. Medical advice should be taken regarding contraception, and should certainly be sought if children are wanted. I am not qualified to discuss pregnancy in paraplegia. However, there are certain dangers and difficulties, similar to those experienced by able-bodied women, but these difficulties are more pronounced, particularly for women with cervical lesions. So I repeat – paraplegics and specifically tetraplegics, should consult a spinal specialist if they plan to have children.

Women with complete lesions, like men, will not experience a normal orgasm. However, many women claim they experience an orgasm through stimulation of other areas of the body, such as their breasts, neck and ears. These areas, known as the erogenous zones, also include the mouth, lips, nipples, the genital areas and insides of thighs. In all these areas or zones, there is a concentration of nerve fibres, making them more sensitive.

There are several possible dangers and practical difficulties for those anticipating intercourse, and special care and consideration will need to be taken by both partners. If the disabled female is a tetraplegic some difficulty may be experienced with her breathing during intercourse, due to the weight of her partner. The able-bodied partner should therefore support part if not all his weight on his elbows or forearms. Over-spastic legs are another problem. It might be necessary to secure them with suitable soft ties. Care should be taken not to tie too tightly, for this can result in skin damage and also fracture of bones. Choice of surface is all important because skin damage and bruising can easily occur.

As with males, females should empty the bladder before intercourse; the risk of retention is less, but quite possible. The prime concern is to prevent the embarrassment of becoming wet. For obvious reasons it would be unwise to attempt intercourse on the night a laxative has been taken.

Where problems persist that prevent good sexual relations, such as over-spastic legs, there is often a simple answer or some treatment available that will help the situation. Therefore advice from a spinal specialist should be sought without hesitation.

Considerable patience, trial and experiment is required before satisfactory relationships can be reached when one partner is paralysed. It must be remembered that when two people are in love, any physical contact that is agreeable between each other is all right. One partner may want to try a certain position for intercourse but the other partner may at first feel awkward and not wish to participate. This is understandable but wrong. Try everything, more than once, until a satisfactory relationship is reached. Many disabled people practise oral sexual relations; some may regard this as unpleasant or crude, but many able-bodied people practise it too. There is nothing physically or mentally wrong with oral sex; it is a healthy contact between two people to be enjoyed. Again there is a positive need to take great care and not forget the probable loss of feeling and the harm that could result.

The involvement of sexual activity in both sexes and its enjoyment is I believe a leading factor in psychological rehabilitation. Because there may be loss of normal sexual outlet through orgasm, this is no reason to assume that sexual drive or desire is also lost. On the contrary, sexual drive and desire remain strong and it is this fact that makes me shudder when the paraplegic or tetraplegic is referred to as impotent.

Young people injured before experiencing intercourse and orgasm, may spend the rest of their lives wondering, while those fortunate enough to have experienced intercourse before injury will have memories. This problem, I believe, often leads many newly disabled to drink more than is good for them, in an attempt to numb the mind to the reality of their situation. Again there is no quick and simple answer and periods of frustration will be experienced. In marriage, as in other close relationships, much of the sexual frustration experienced is more easily expelled by seeing sexual satisfaction and happiness in the able-bodied partner.

A little research into sexual diversion through viewing erotic material, books, films etc., is being carried out mainly in the U.S.A. This might be of some help in the future, but to date the results are vague. Further research into sexual problems of disabled people of all kinds has been, and still is being, conducted by The National Fund for Research into Crippling Diseases – the project being carried out by the Research Institute for Consumer Affairs (Sex and the Physically Handicapped).

PROSTHETIC DEVICES

It is possible to obtain many prosthetic devices, or marital aids, which in certain circumstances can be of great help and benefit to disabled people. Many aids can be regarded as nothing more than sex toys. Others have been designed under medical supervision to cater especially for disabilities of all kinds. Should people wish to try using any of these aids, then an open mind must be adopted and continual trials made.

Such aids include an artificial penis that can be strapped on when it has been impossible for the male to obtain an erection. Another type of artificial penis available is of hollow construction into which an actual penis can be inserted and held by an inflatable balloon device. This is useful when only a partial erection can be obtained. There is also a hand held penis, a 'Dildo', which can be used in the hand by either partner. Should patients wish to try an artificial penis, a lubricant such as KY jelly or Johnson's baby oil should be used. This might also be of help under normal circumstances. Petroleum jelly should not be used.

There are many and various types of vibrators designed to

stimulate males and females. All these items can be studied by obtaining catalogues. Addresses of suppliers can be found in most magazines of an erotic nature or by contacting one of the many sex shops.

7

Physiotherapy

Physiotherapy plays a major role throughout the whole treatment of the paraplegic and it is aimed at strengthening and maintaining the body in the best possible condition to provide maximum independence and confidence. Early treatment consists mainly of daily passive movements to all paralysed limbs, thus maintaining a full range of movement, and preventing contractures and stiffness of joints. Electro-therapy is sometimes given to stimulate weak muscles and keep nerve pathways open. Breathing exercises and chest physiotherapy are often required to treat or prevent chest complications, particularly for patients with cervical and high thoracic lesions.

At the stage of active rehabilitation patients are taught to strengthen their remaining muscles through exercises, weight lifting, and springs and pulleys. They are also taught balance control sitting on a plinth in front of a mirror, by using muscles of the trunk and neck to compensate for loss of leg and other movement. This trains them to sit in the wheelchair without losing balance, and leaving their hands and arms free.

Training will also include techniques of transferring from wheelchair to bed, to car, on and off the lavatory and from the ground to chair, standing with leg plasters or calipers as required and where possible, walking with the aid of crutches or walking sticks. Patients will learn all these skills as normal routine treatment. I therefore do not intend to go into details but would just emphasize some points and stress the benefits of continuing treatment after discharge from hospital.

PASSIVE MOVEMENTS

These should be continued to all paralysed limbs at regular and frequent intervals. Not only does this maintain the full range of movement, it helps maintain a good circulation, which is so important in preventing pressure sores. They are also valuable from the cosmetic approach, in that they help in the prevention of deformed and contracted hands. These are often seen in old patients with cervical lesions and can be unsightly and difficult to manage.

STANDING

This is a most beneficial part of treatment and should be practised as often as possible. Many patients become lazy about standing, and forget the benefits which include better drainage of the urinary system, thus aiding prevention of infection and formation of stones, and the weight-bearing which helps to prevent bones becoming brittle (osteoporosis). Standing helps also with the prevention of contractures to hips, knees and ankles and in particular 'foot drop' – the contraction of the Achilles tendon, which prevents the foot lying flat on the floor. It reduces spasms, improves circulation and prevents sores. Standing gives a general effect of well-being, and boosts morale in being able to talk to others at the same standing level, and is a good form of exercise!

PREVENTION OF CHEST COMPLICATIONS

The prevention of chest infection is all important. This is more difficult for patients with high lesions who are unable to expand their lungs as normal. Regular daily deep breathing exercises will help maintain the lung tissue in the best possible condition. Regular changes of position, turns in bed, standing and leaning forward in the wheelchair all aid the lungs to drain naturally. During the summer months, as much time as possible should

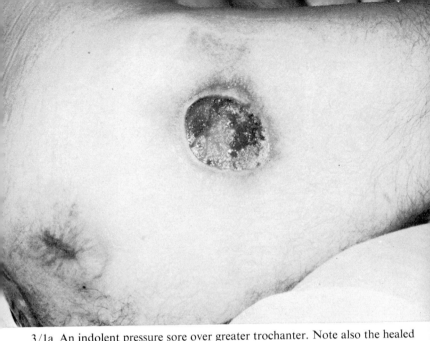

3/1a An indolent pressure sore over greater trochanter. Note also the healed sore posteriorly.

3/1b The same sore as in 3/1a now healed after all pressure had been relieved.

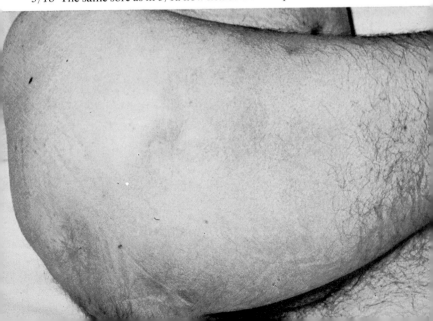

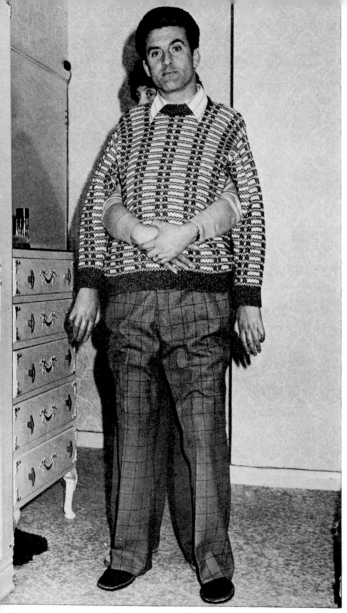

3/2 The author, a C4 lesion, standing; the support is from his wife—note the position of her hands. Leg extension is maintained by wearing plaster splints.

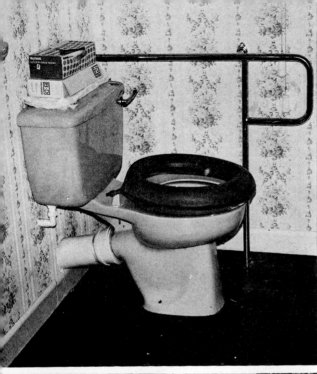

4/1 Inflatable lavatory seat, which will fit over a normal lavatory seat.

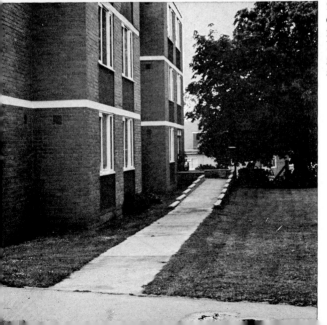

9/1 Ramped entrance to house from pavement. Note the long gradual incline and side walls.

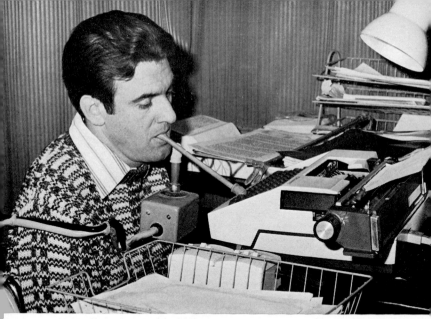

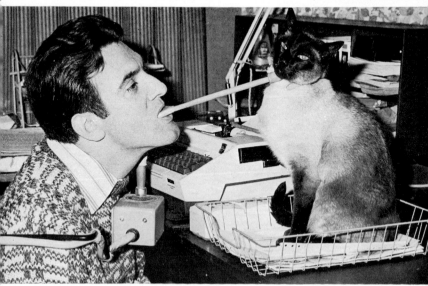

8/1 The author typing, using an electric typewriter and a mouth stick. Note also the chin operated control for the wheelchair.

8/2 Bliss!

be spent in the fresh air and will be beneficial to the lungs. During the winter months, try and avoid going out unnecessarily, stay in the warm and avoid mixing with people known to have a cough or cold.

Where a chest infection is suspected, a doctor must be consulted immediately, particularly with cervical lesions. Difficulty with breathing may require hospital treatment. Sore throats and head colds should not be ignored and often a day or two spent in bed with a cold will prevent the infection travelling to the chest. Some patients may find difficulty in breathing through their nose. The cause is sometimes attributable to the spinal cord injury and the disturbance of the nervous system. This condition known as Horner's syndrome has many effects, one being blockage of the nasal passages called 'Guttmann's sign'. Should this persist, consult your doctor who may prescribe decongestant drops or spray.

CHEST CARE

Good understanding of chest care is most important, particularly for patients with cervical and high thoracic lesions. These patients will have paralysis of abdominal and chest muscles resulting in an inability to cough normally. Because of this, chest infection and the inhaling of food and drink can be fatal. Our lungs are made in such a way that it is normal for the tissue to produce mucus. This keeps the linings of the delicate tubes moist and clean to allow the exchange of oxygen with the blood when we breathe. Mucus is produced in little tubes known as bronchioles. Lining these tubes are tiny appendages, like little hairs (the cilia), that are constantly on the move carrying mucus through the lungs until it eventually reaches the throat. At this point an automatic reflex is triggered and we cough to 'clear the throat'.

With high lesions this reflex is still present, but due to paralysis of chest and abdominal muscles it is not possible to cough mucus up in the normal manner. Any irritation tends to cause the person to inhale sharply thus drawing mucus back into the lungs which is followed by an attack of choking. When this happens, assistance is usually required to cough and keep the throat and lungs clear.

ASSISTED COUGHING

Assisted coughing is a method of helping the patient to react as he would if his chest and abdominal muscles were working normally. Coughing is simply the forcing of air out of the lungs under pressure. As the air is expelled, it takes any foreign matter with it. Nature's way of doing this is for the abdominal muscles to force the diaphragm upwards. At the same time the chest muscles (the intercostals), contract the rib-cage thus forcing air out of the lungs under pressure. When these muscles are paralysed it is necessary to mimic nature by applying external pressure over the rib-cage. This is done by an assistant placing hands on either side of the chest and as the paralysed person exhales squeezing the chest. Care has to be taken not to squeeze too hard for fear of damaging the ribs.

An alternative method is to place hands over the abdominal muscles and as the paralysed person exhales, push inwards and upwards. The diaphragm is thus pushed upwards forcing air out of the lungs. Both methods of assisted coughing require practice, the former method I feel is the more satisfactory, because there is no danger of hurting the stomach.

Experience soon teaches patients how to keep their throats clear by trick coughing techniques, combining a weak cough, exhaling of air and contractions of the throat. By coughing before mucus can start an irritation and choking attack, more often than not the normal lung excretions can be cleared without assistance. When irritation is caused by infection or smoking, assistance will certainly be required to keep air-ways clear.

Smoking

Smoking is a classic example of unnecessary irritation causing the formation of an excess of mucus. Not only does smoke cause the lungs to produce more mucus, but nicotine in tobacco stops the movement of the cilia – the little hairs – that carry mucus along the tubes of the lungs.

Smoking therefore causes two immediate problems: the formation of an excess of mucus, and the prevention of nature's own method of cleaning and lubricating the lungs. This then results in blockage of the bronchioles which may become infected and lead to a shortage of oxygen, which causes breathlessness and chronic bronchitis.

An able-bodied person with the normal coughing mechanism can overcome the problem of an excess of mucus caused through smoking, by forcing it out of their lungs under increased pressure. This is generated through violent coughing which in turn will cause damage to the lungs over a number of years. The paralysed person who continues to smoke will be plagued by chest problems leading to chronic lung conditions. The short and simple answer is that nobody *should* smoke and patients with high lesions should *never* smoke.

8

Return to the Community

DISCHARGE FROM HOSPITAL

Besides the physical and mental turmoil that paraplegics often experience during their very long periods of care and protection under hospital conditions, final discharge back into the community can be and often is, as traumatic as the day when they were first admitted to hospital. Although most patients will have spent progressively longer periods at home prior to discharge, it is not until they are finally on their own that the true impact of everything that has happened during the preceding months really registers with dramatic clarity.

In the previous chapters I have outlined some of the psychological and physical difficulties associated with the immediate effect of a spinal cord injury. I have also supplied guidelines directed towards good physical care for the future. The importance and value of all the information provided may not register for a long time. Readers might well wonder how they can manage to prevent or avoid some of the complications mentioned. The most positive, effective, and probably the only way of doing this is to aim to remember the points I have stressed and try hard and conscientiously to live by the rules. I would not be truthful if I were to say there are no inevitable complications to paralysis. There are and everybody will, from time to time, experience problems, some minor and some more serious. One thing is certain; if patients do not try and live their lives within the rules, then they will be inviting problems.

This is sometimes difficult to understand immediately. For

after discharge there is an automatic tendency to try and resume life as it was before the onset of paralysis. A normal enough reaction; but whereas the mind might be anxious and willing to do this, the body is not always able to cope. I am not saying one cannot enjoy life to the full. On the contrary, a vast majority of paraplegics and tetraplegics live very full, happy and contented lives and are fine examples to many able-bodied people. Nevertheless it will take time to re-adjust to a new code of living and time to develop a natural balance between mind and body.

Depending on domestic circumstances, final discharge may be either to the patient's own home, to institutional care, such as Cheshire Homes or Young Disabled Units, or to a rehabilitation or job retraining centre. Regardless of where patients are discharged, a sense of fear and apprehension is often experienced. Tetraplegics who are totally unable to fend for themselves are frequently quite terrified that institutional staff or relatives will not be able to care for them in the manner to which they have become accustomed.

To fortify patients over this disturbing initial discharge period, staff and relatives should constantly offer comfort and reassurance and remain consistently even-tempered for as long as it takes the disabled individual to settle down.

It is my opinion that however long patients initially spend in hospital following injury, they will not psychologically adjust to their new circumstances for at least 12 months after discharge. This is equally true from the physical aspect: merely experiencing the effects of living outside hospital through all the changes of the seasons in a wheelchair is sufficient in itself to prove my point.

Those fortunate enough to be discharged back to their old home, or even a new one, will it is hoped have had sufficient basic entrance and doorway adaptations carried out before their return at least to give them reasonable access. Sadly, this is not always the case because it does appear that medical rehabilitation works faster than social integration! It is impossible to describe how individuals of all ages and from all walks of life, manage to rehabilitate after their discharge. The majority do settle into their new life-style after a reasonable period of time, particularly those who return to employment of one kind or another. Alas, there is always an unfortunate minority of patients, often young, sometimes depressed and carrying a 'chip on the shoulder' complex who find great difficulty in facing up to life from a wheelchair.

These people seem to have lost all sense of responsibility. They waste their days away sitting in front of a television, backing horses, drinking far too much alcohol or by just looking out of the window. Exactly why some people react in this way would be excellent material for a behavioural psychologist to study. Obviously they have not come to terms with their disability for one of many possible reasons.

Some paraplegics admit that massive compensation settlements and social security benefits take away their incentive to work. This might well be right up to a point, for this financial security does provide people with a means to live without working. I am not necessarily suggesting that people should seek employment at this stage, but I do maintain that a temporary occupation will stimulate their brains and prevent them from vegetating. If at a later stage they should wish to seek more lasting and satisfying employment, and circumstances permit, so much the better. By occupying the brain, there is less opportunity to think about disability and gradually the mental anguish becomes less.

Undoubtedly domestic circumstances have a large bearing on people's activities. In institutional surroundings it is not always easy to follow an occupation of one's own choice, for the whole Home has to be considered. Happily however, many of these establishments are most understanding and free and easy in their outlook. If a patient is in receipt of social security benefits, there are perhaps limitations to the amount he or she is allowed to earn. But there can be no limitation on the amount of occupational therapy undertaken, the more the merrier!

I have often been asked what it was that motivated and inspired me back to life. Likewise I have asked many others the same question. The conclusion reached is that it is not just one thing in particular that may happen on a certain day, but a series of events and circumstances that accumulate over an unpredictable period (Plate 8/1 and 8/2).

The initial key and responsibility for motivation lies squarely in the hands of the medical and paramedical staff. These are the experts who initially undertake the task of restoring the patient to the best possible physical and mental condition. As part of that treatment they are pledged to create the correct atmosphere for patients to relearn that life is still worth living despite the severity of the disability.

As the medical consultant leads the team, he is the one who should direct and demonstrate the style of treatment. This is usually achieved through regular ward teaching rounds, when individual capabilities and achievements of patients are discussed. Much of this information will be intentionally overheard by other patients and staff thus encouraging them to do the same or even better. Ward Sisters who maintain a happy, efficient, progressive manner, do much to instil enthusiasm and if one vital word can describe what it is that motivates anybody to do anything, then it must be enthusiasm. The enthusiasm exhibited by all members of a medical and paramedical team working closely with patients, will create a little spark of motivation in the patients' hearts by the time they are ready for discharge.

This is only the start; motivation must come from within and as I have said will depend largely on domestic circumstances. It is quite understandable for someone to become withdrawn, depressed and disinterested in everything life can offer if, for example, he has been rejected by family and friends and packed off to an institutional home full of strangers. Where an atmosphere of love and caring exists and the disabled person is made to feel wanted, he will then respond by wanting to give all he can in return, encouraged by a purpose for living and a reason to make something of life. The desire to be wanted is by no means exclusive to the disabled. It applies equally to people in all walks of life. A disabled person has to cope with the extra burdens and frustrations of fighting his disability, and so it is vitally important for him to receive support and encouragement in his endless struggle.

There are many organizations and charities well equipped and experienced to help disabled people rediscover themselves, by providing information and guidance (see p. 152).

Besides the many charitable organizations willing to help the disabled, the Department of Health and Social Security can offer a very wide range of practical help in the form of family doctor and hospital services, aids and equipment, financial benefits, and help from local authority social services. Much of the Department's help is obscure and patients will experience difficulty in obtaining facts. There is a Department of Health booklet entitled *Help for Handicapped People* No. HB1 and all disabled people should obtain a copy.

Every disabled person should purchase a copy of the *Chronically Sick and Disabled Persons Act 1970*. This can be bought from Her Majesty's Stationery Office and outlines disabled persons' entitlements under the law. This Act, broadly speaking, is an extension of the 1948 National Assistance Act and when sections apply to local social services in particular, they tend to interpret the Act according to their circumstances. Consequently this leads to considerable variance in the help provided from area to area. In order to ensure that disabled people receive adequate help, social service officials frequently subject applicants to means tests before their requests are considered. H.M.S.O. addresses are given on p. 161.

MEDICAL CHECK-UPS

Regardless of how much patients hate the thought of re-entering hospital, even as outpatients, it is vital to have regular check-ups. This cannot be stressed enough. Often underlying complications exist without a patient feeling the slightest effect. Such complications, if discovered in time, can often be treated without subjecting patients to too much inconvenience, but if they are left until permanent damage is done, then patients must not expect hospital staff to perform miracles.

Check-ups or follow-up care consist of a blood test, a urine test, a neurological examination, a physical examination and occasionally an I.V.P. The latter is a series of X-rays lasting about 30 minutes to determine kidney function and the efficiency of the remainder of the urinary system.

The responsibility for having a check-up rests in patients' own hands. Arrangements should be made through their general practitioner. Patients will be advised by their spinal specialist about the need for regular I.V.Ps. I.V.Ps. are expensive and are not carried out unnecessarily, so if you are told to have one at a certain time, do not miss the opportunity. I.V.Ps. can be given at all large hospitals. Unless there are special reasons it is not necessary to return to a spinal unit for one, although this may be more satisfactory. Six-monthly blood and urine tests should be carried out and these can be arranged at any hospital. Patients naturally depend heavily on special spinal units for their treatment. This is understandable for only a few general hospitals are staffed and equipped to cater for the needs of paraplegia. However, most can cope with routine check-up examinations and they would refer patients back to a spinal unit if in doubt, or if treatment were required.

It is every patient's duty to encourage their family doctor to take an interest in their condition and not bypass him by going directly to a specialized centre. Family doctors should be kept informed about what is going on, so that they may refer patients back to a spinal specialist if necessary.

GENERAL HYGIENE

Personal hygiene is all important in the daily battle to prevent complications. Very often regular washing of paralysed limbs is forgotten. A complete bath weekly, plus the daily washing of groins and bottom is the minimum. This will keep skin free of dry patches and is usually sufficient to prevent septic spots. Many choose to shave pubic hair, and this certainly prevents the collection of skin adhesive where condom urinals are worn. It also reduces infection, particularly for those requiring indwelling catheters.

Particular attention should be paid to the care of feet. The formation of dry, hard skin on the feet is a common problem, and one which can be controlled by regular soaking and washing in warm soapy water. If it persists, the regular application of lanolin ointment after washing will help prevent further formation. Toe and finger nails often become hard and brittle and these should be kept cut short. Toe nails often grow inwards and become infected, and this is a cause of increased spasms. Should this problem persist, it might be necessary to have them removed, so consult your doctor or district nurse.

Teeth are of particular importance to tetraplegics, who depend heavily on them for holding various things. Remember to take good care of them. Once they have gone, false teeth cannot do the work of real ones. Have regular six-monthly check-ups with your dentist.

Hygiene also applies to clothing. Soiled clothes will cause endless skin problems, irritations, rashes and spots. Cushion covers and sheepskins require regular washing otherwise they become hard and matted and another cause of sores and infection. Bedclothing can be a source of skin problems. Sheets and pillowcases should be changed at regular and frequent intervals. If pillows are used to lie on, whenever possible these should be thoroughly aired in direct sunlight.

WEIGHT AND DIET

In an attempt to keep their weight down, paraplegics should, unless guided otherwise, aim to eat mostly protein and roughage. Carbohydrates such as bread or potatoes should be kept to the minimum. This is sometimes very difficult, for with the present price of food, particularly high protein foods, and coupled with the inability to exercise normally, it is very easy to eat the wrong foods and put on weight.

Excessive weight is difficult to lose and life automatically becomes harder for the individual to manage. An over-weight tetraplegic, dependent on assistance, can make life impossible for families, district nurses and others who have to attend them. This often leads to the necessity of moving paraplegics into homes and the break up of happy family circles.

There is only one way of preventing excessive weight and that is to restrict the intake of food and drink (not water). Try to match the quantity you eat by the amount of exercise taken. For example, a C6 complete lesion would require roughly 1400 calories a day. With limited movement, it is impossible to burn off more energy than that.

People vary in how much they can eat and how much weight they put on. It is impossible to lay down rules, and common sense has to be applied. If problems of over-weight do exist, patients should discuss the situation with their doctor who can call upon the help of a dietician.

THE GENERAL PRACTITIONER

One of the very first things a patient should do after discharge from hospital, is to register with a general practitioner. A list of general practitioners can be found in the local post office of the area in which you are living. Should you have difficulty in finding a doctor, you should contact your local Family Practitioner Committee, whose address will also be found at the post office or Citizens' Advice Bureau. Patients are advised to ask their doctor to see them immediately after they are discharged, when they are fit and well, because he may not have seen a paraplegic person before. The doctor will then have a basis for comparison to work on should he be called at other times.

It is the policy of spinal units to teach paraplegics as much as they can absorb about their own management. This is essential to survival after discharge, and consequently patients sometimes know more about themselves than their family doctor. In these circumstances it can be difficult to converse with the family doctor as the patient instinctively dictates treatment previously recommended in hospital. Patients should exercise tact and discretion and perhaps suggest to their doctor that they have read about such treatment in publications about paraplegia. If that fails it can always be diplomatically suggested to your doctor that he telephones the consultant who looked after you in the spinal unit or hospital. But discharged patients must always be on their guard against ignorance about paraplegia and its latest forms of treatment. It is still something of a Cinderella condition to many general practitioners who frankly admit they have little or no knowledge and experience of handling it. If this situation exists in your case it may be advisable to change your local doctor.

PRESCRIPTION CHARGES

Certain groups of people do not have to pay prescription charges. These include children under 15 and adults over 65. Exemption also includes people with continuing physical disabilities. Leaflet EC 91 *General Information on Exemptions and Refunds* from social security offices will describe how to go about obtaining an exemption certificate.

9

Housing and Living

LOCAL AUTHORITY SOCIAL AND HEALTH SERVICES

Local authorities are empowered to provide care for the disabled as laid down in the *Chronically Sick and Disabled Persons Act 1970*. In theory it is incumbent on the authority to meet the need. The assessment of need lies entirely within the authority's discretion and will inevitably vary from area to area.

Section 2 of the Chronically Sick and Disabled Persons Act
Provision of welfare services. 1948 c. 29
2. (1) Where a local authority having functions under Section 29 of the National Assistance Act 1948 are satisfied in the case of any person to whom that section applies who is ordinarily resident in their area that it is necessary in order to meet the needs of that person for that authority to make arrangements for all or any of the following matters, namely
a) the provision of practical assistance for that person in his home;
b) the provision for that person of, or assistance to that person in obtaining, wireless, television, library or similar recreational facilities;
c) the provision for that person of lectures, games, outings or other recreational facilities outside his home or assistance to that person in taking advantage of educational facilities available to him;
d) the provision for that person of facilities for, or assistance in, travelling to and from his home for the purpose of participating in any services provided under arrangements

made by the authority under the said Section 29 or, with the approval of the authority, in any services provided otherwise than as aforesaid which are similar to services which could be provided under such arrangements;

e) the provision of assistance for that person in arranging for the carrying out of any works of adaptation in his home or the provision of any additional facilities designed to secure his greater safety, comfort or convenience;

f) facilitating the taking of holidays by that person, whether at holiday homes or otherwise and whether provided under arrangements made by the authority or otherwise;

g) the provision of meals for that person whether in his home or elsewhere;

h) the provision for that person of, or assistance to that person in obtaining, a telephone and any special equipment necessary to enable him to use a telephone,

then, notwithstanding anything in any scheme made by the authority under the said Section 29, but subject to the provisions of section 35 (2) of that Act (which requires local authorities to exercise their functions under Part III of that Act under the general guidance of the Secretary of State and in accordance with the provisions of any regulations made for the purpose), it shall be the duty of that authority to make those arrangements in exercise of their functions under the said Section 29.

SOCIAL WORKERS

Generally speaking social workers employed outside special spinal units, lack general knowledge regarding the needs of paraplegics. It has been my experience that one of the solutions to this weak link in the rehabilitation chain is for patients and their relatives to find out for themselves what is available. This information will include facts about the social services, and how they can be applied to individual requirements.

At varying periods of time after a patient is admitted to a spinal unit, the hospital-based social worker will interview both patient and relatives in an attempt to assess their domestic circumstances in relation to the subsequent return home of the paraplegic, possibly in a wheelchair. After this initial meeting, when items such as suitability of housing are discussed, the hospital-based social worker usually writes to the social services department in the patient's own home area, outlining the general situation and arranging a possible visit to the patient's home. This visit is either carried out by the hospital social worker and occupational therapist, or by the community social worker and domiciliary occupational therapist and perhaps the district nurse. After the patient's home has been carefully assessed regarding suitability for wheelchair access, and lavatories, bathroom, bedroom, kitchen and living room have been considered, certain recommendations are put forward to both the patient's family and the local authority.

These recommendations will vary depending primarily on whether the property in question is privately or council-owned. If it is rented from the local council, recommendations will be made to the local housing authority either for necessary alterations and adaptations to be made under *Section 2 of the Chronically Sick and Disabled Persons Act*, or for the disabled person and his family to be rehoused in a more suitable house or bungalow, or for a purpose-built bungalow suitable in every aspect to the disabled person's needs to be provided. This latter will only happen in a minority of cases. The extent to which local authorities are willing to co-operate under Section 2 of the Act varies considerably from one area to another and basically depends on local finances.

When the property in question is privately owned, either by the patient or the family, or if it is owned by a landlord and rented, the question of alteration or adaptation is a very different matter. The first consideration to be taken into account is suitability and whether it is a practical proposition to either alter or adapt the property. Many old houses with steps and stairs all over the place are not worth modifying to suit a wheelchair. The second consideration is cost.

If the property is totally unsuitable; and this is for patients and their families to decide, regardless of what the social services may say or think; or if the owner or landlord refused to allow alterations, there are two alternatives: to buy or rent another more suitable house, flat or bungalow, or to apply to the local housing authority for a suitable council owned property. Whichever option is taken obviously depends on personal, domestic and financial circumstances. It is often very much quicker and certainly more satisfactory to move into a new privately owned property, rather than rely on the local council to find suitable council owned accommodation.

If the privately owned property is found to be suitable, providing suggested alterations are made to accommodate a wheelchair, then the question arises of costs and who is going to pay. Under Section 2 of the *Chronically Sick and Disabled Persons Act*, local authorities will make all necessary alterations and adaptations to property to house a disabled person who qualifies under the Act. There is no reference as to whether the property is privately or council owned. Unfortunately social service departments interpret the Act as being an extension of the 1948 *National Assistance Act*, which gives them the power to subject applicants for help under the *Chronically Sick and Disabled Persons Act*, to a means test.

I doubt very much if there are many people who would turn to the social services for financial help with house alterations if they could genuinely afford to pay themselves. It is often the average family who are already sacrificing a great deal paying off a house mortgage or paying for their children's education, who, when distressed and not knowing which way to turn next, suddenly find themselves subjected to the humiliation of a means test. Authorities maintain that the means test is the only way of ensuring that help is distributed fairly, yet not all applicants are subjected to such a test. Perhaps in time to come a more efficient method of assessing genuine need will evolve other than the obvious physical needs of paraplegia.

HOUSE ALTERATIONS

Property, whether private or council owned, should, whenever possible, be suitably adapted or modified **before** paraplegics are finally discharged from hospital. Not only would this seem common sense for the benefit of the disabled person, it is also vitally important to give families as a whole every possible support in the often difficult task they are undertaking – that of caring for their disabled relative. Only too often one hears of families and marriages breaking up, which can be attributed to unsuitable housing primarily, and to inadequate help and advice.

I think most people would agree that a ground floor flat or bungalow type of accommodation is most suitable for a wheelchair user. Many wheelchair users do live in ordinary houses and blocks of flats that have been fitted with lifts, and it may prove less expensive to provide this type of alteration to a house, rather than rehousing the whole family.

Obvious disadvantages of lifts are the risks of mechanical failure, power-cuts, fire, vandalism and difficulty in operation for the more severely disabled, together with the loss of space and major alterations necessary. However, there are many firms providing house alterations of this nature which seem to be most satisfactory; some even provide external lifts (see Appendix).

The most important consideration when assessing whether a property is suitable for a wheelchair user is that of easy access. This means that the person in the wheelchair should be able to enter and leave the property without assistance. It also includes easy access to and from the road, and frequently necessitates the construction of a ramp in place of steps and a suitable concrete pathway. Ramps should be of concrete construction; wooden ramps can burn, be removed and are often slippery. Ramps should be gradual and wide enough for safety purposes and if possible constructed with side walls and rails (Plate 9/1).

Whenever possible a property with at least two suitable entrances should be chosen. Ramps may be necessary and I do not feel it is unreasonable to ask the Social Services Department to provide these under the terms of the *Chronically Sick and Disabled Persons Act*. Should they be reluctant to provide a ramp, then you may need to go to the extreme of suggesting that you will hold them legally responsible for your safety in the event of fire!

All doors, including the main entrance, should be sufficiently wide to allow free access, eliminating the risk of damaging hands. This usually means that doors will require alteration to make them approximately 90cm (3ft) wide. Internal doors of the sliding type are in most cases more suitable. Front doors that open inwards may be difficult for the wheelchair user to close on leaving the property. Sometimes the addition of a D-shape handle fixed to the centre of the door permits the paraplegic to reach back and pull the door shut. Locks and latches may also require alteration, such as lowering them for easy reach.

Specific alterations and modifications will vary enormously depending upon the layout of the accommodation. Obviously all steps should be removed and replaced by ramps. Inside these can be of wooden construction, providing they are fixed securely. Electric light switches may require to be lowered and socket plugs raised to 3 feet from the floor.

Whenever possible a lavatory and bathroom should be accessible from the bedroom and at least one other lavatory provided for other members of the household to use. Conventional bath tubs may be difficult to get in and out of and a shower unit might prove more satisfactory. This of course is a personal choice. There are firms who produce specially designed shower units with the disabled in mind. Most such units require the user to transfer out of the wheelchair onto a fitted seat within the unit, which can often prove awkward. Where plenty of space is available, an open tiled and drained area with shower above, when the paraplegic can sit in a shower-chair fitted with foot-rests, is so much more satisfactory.

Reconstruction of a kitchen, especially for the disabled house-wife, is a very important aspect. Not only must the kitchen be functional, space is of paramount importance. Split level cooker units are most practical, where the oven opens just above knee level. Some paraplegic housewives prefer oven doors that hinge downwards, they can then rest whatever they are cooking on the door. Others say the door that hinges down prevents them getting close enough to put pots and pans into the oven, they prefer the side-hinged door. Again this is a personal choice. Naturally all cupboards must be accessible from the sitting position. The washing-up sink unit must be placed to allow the knees and wheelchair underneath. Waste and supply water pipes should be well lagged to prevent burns to knees.

Kitchen modification for a tetraplegic is even more crucial and great thought must be put into every aspect of design. Unless the tetraplegic has use of tricep muscles (the muscle which straightens the arm), the risk of trying to cook, handling boiling hot pots and pans, should be carefully considered. I suggest that all tetraplegics and especially those without triceps, stick to handling cold food and drink.

Adequate heating is another important consideration when altering or building a house. Living in the British Isles central heating is almost essential. The choice of system will depend on circumstances, but with the everlasting rise in fuel costs, anybody installing a new heating system would be wise to consider the addition of solar panels! If open fires are used, care should be taken to ensure that coals do not fall from the grate and that the wheelchair user does not sit too close and possibly burn his legs.

Special adaptations, modifications and aids may be necessary for paraplegic children. Examples of equipment available include variable height wash-basins that have telescopic drain-pipes. As the child grows the basin can be raised on adjustable brackets. Inserts for toilet seats can be fitted over the standard size toilet seat, thus leaving the toilet basically unaltered. Further examples of these aids and others which help towards greater independence within a house, together with ideal modifications and layouts of kitchens, bathrooms, bedrooms, and electrical equipment are all splendidly displayed in the Disabled Living Foundation. The Foundation also provide an up-to-date information service on practically everything connected with disablement of all kinds.

In theory all housing alterations and adaptations should be provided for under Section 2 of the *Chronically Sick and Disabled Persons Act*. In practice this does not always happen, for some social service departments are only able to provide a bare minimum; some are more generous. Some provide interest-free loans to house owners to make their own alterations. The degree of help that one can expect to receive appears to depend on where you live, how determined you can be and the extent of your problem.

Personal note

I strongly urge anybody experiencing difficulties in obtaining what they feel is their entitlement not to give in easily, but to seek advice, help and assistance from organizations experienced in dealing with these issues (see Appendix). This is by no means a biased view directed towards the social services, it is merely my wish that patients and their families should receive that to which they are entitled. Time and again some social services departments will refuse requests because they themselves do not accurately interpret the many complicated rules and regulations laid down regarding these matters.

It should also be made perfectly clear that in no way are patients compelled to involve social service departments in their domestic affairs and rehabilitation. Many people enter and leave hospital managing their own affairs. However the majority of paraplegics are compelled to rely on the system for at least some degree of assistance, usually because of financial limitations.

Before final discharge and usually about the time patients are ready to go home for weekends, application is made by the hospital authorities to the local social services for home nursing aids and equipment. These aids are basic requirements for survival at home and are supplied, if required, regardless of circumstances. After final discharge, if further aids are required, these can be obtained through the district nurse or social worker.

BEDS

It is of prime importance for a paraplegic to have a suitable bed (see p. 42). Social services departments are able to supply many different types for patients requiring a bed of the hospital sort.

Spinal units generally suggest that paraplegics sleep on a sorbo-rubber mattress at least 10cm (4in) thick. This is the standard type used on the old-fashioned hospital bed. More modern hospital beds that can be supplied to patients are equipped with features such as a variable height adjustment, which is of great value in transferring. A visit to the Disabled Living Foundation will give patients the opportunity of seeing and trying the many different beds available. One particular bed in use and on issue to patients in their own homes is the King's Fund Bed. This is variable in height and can be fitted with a monkey-pole if so required.

In extreme cases where a patient is very large and heavy to turn, or having problems with pressure sores, the Stoke Mandeville Egerton electric turning bed can be supplied. This is usually on the recommendation of a hospital consultant or general practitioner. These beds are very large and would certainly require a big bedroom.

Many patients do not need to borrow a bed from the social services department, because they find their own beds are quite satisfactory. Provided no problems are experienced regarding pressure, an ordinary bed with a good interior spring mattress is quite acceptable and often more comfortable.

Ripple-mattress

Whereas the majority of patients sleep on standard types of mattresses and train themselves to wake and turn over every 3 or 4 hours many paraplegics and tetraplegics have difficulty in turning themselves. Rather than call for help during the night, they sleep on a ripple-mattress which is placed on top of either a sorbo-rubber or spring-interior mattress.

The ripple-mattress, manufactured by the same company as the ripple-cushion, has proved to be of great value to many paralysed and elderly people who are unable to turn themselves during the night. Again it must be remembered that this mattress is only an aid in the prevention of pressure sores and where individuals concerned are able to turn themselves at regular intervals, they should be instructed to do so rather than depend on mechanical aids.

The ripple-mattress works on the same principle as the seat-cushion, although the tubular sections are larger and the electric-operating pump is mains powered. (This should be remembered in the event of power failures.) The ripple-mattress is available on loan from local social services. Most patients requiring them will have the loan arranged before leaving hospital. Otherwise they should speak with their general practitioner, district nurse or social worker who will then make the necessary arrangements to obtain one. Those who have become dependent on the ripple-mattress, should always remember to take it with them on holidays or if they are admitted to hospital. For emergency use, those who can afford to purchase a spare mattress and pump are advised to do so.

Hoists

In many cases, particularly when the patient is very heavy or spastic, it may be necessary for relatives or attendants to use a hoist to transfer the patient in and out of their chair, bed, bath or car.

There are many different makes available, either mechanically, hydraulically or electrically operated. Choice of type will depend on circumstances. Many disabled people are able to live on their own with the aid of an electrically operated hoist such as the Wessex. This hoist can be fitted to an overhead rail system for carrying the patient suspended, from bathroom to bedroom for example. Other smaller mechanical or hydraulically operated hoists can be wheeled from one room to another with patients suspended from them which is useful for getting in and out of the bath and returning to bed. These require an attendant to operate them. Another hoist, produced by Birvill & Son, Primrose Road, Hersham, Walton-on-Thames, Surrey, can be fixed to the roof of a car for lifting patients in and out.

There are no hard and fast rules regarding the type of hoist, other than those using a sling. The correct sling should be of the one-piece hammock type. The two-piece sling is dangerous, in case the patient who might be unable to hold on, may spasm and fall out. The inherent disadvantage of the one-piece hammock sling is that on being lowered into the wheelchair it is necessary to leave the sling under the buttocks, tucking it around the sides of the cushion. Users tell me that this causes no problem.

Patients requiring a hoist should contact their local social services or district nurse, who will then make the necessary arrangements to obtain a suitable model. Those requiring hoists before going home will have them supplied by arrangements made through the hospital authorities. The Disabled Living Foundation display many hoists, ready for patients and relatives to try.

Commodes and shower-chairs

In circumstances where toilets are inaccessible, or when there is difficulty in using a lavatory, many paraplegics find that a commode chair in the bedroom or bathroom is of great benefit. Some of these commode chairs can also be used as shower chairs, such as the one produced by Everest & Jennings. These may be more satisfactory than the normal shower-chairs which often have no footrests making it difficult for those with spasms.

Commodes are available through the social services and further information about them can be obtained from the Disabled Living Foundation.

DISTRICT NURSE SERVICE

There are many paraplegics living successfully at home with help from a district nurse. Without the nurse's help they would certainly have to be admitted to hospital or institutional care. Prior to discharge, patients and families who consider they will need help from a district nurse, either on a permanent or temporary basis, can have the service arranged in advance by the hospital nursing authorities. In many cases a district nurse will visit patients in hospital before final discharge, to receive instruction regarding their future care. A district nurse may also visit patients in their homes during a weekend before final discharge to assess the degree of disability and suggest further aids and equipment required to make her job less difficult while making life for the patient more manageable.

There is a heavy demand in most areas for the district nursing service, not only from paraplegics, but from elderly people, heart cases, diabetics, postoperative cases and nursing mothers. All require help. Consequently, it is not always possible for the nurse to attend patients at regular hours. This sometimes makes it difficult to undertake regular employment and keep appointments outside the home.

District nurses are more usually requested by tetraplegics and will undertake all nursing duties such as bladder and bowel management, washing and dressing, treatment of sores and injections. Patients who normally manage without help from the district nursing service and then suddenly find they require assistance (perhaps during a period when they themselves or their attendant are ill), should contact their general practitioner who will then make necessary arrangements.

Services provided by the district nurse vary from area to area and often depend on the type of general practice to which they are attached. There are nurses who will undertake the task of supplying patients with such items as paper sheets and incontinence rolls. Some will bring drugs and medications from the doctor's surgery but others will leave these things for patients to arrange themselves. It is therefore impossible to generalize on the degree of help available.

LAUNDRY SERVICE

In certain circumstances, local authorities may provide a laundry service. Invariably this service is provided for female paraplegics, who, due to the lack of a suitable urine collection device, soil a large amount of personal and bed clothing. Consequently social services departments frequently provide assistance in the form of either a spin or tumble dryer and sometimes a clothes washing machine. Further information regarding the help available in certain areas can be obtained from local social services departments.

HOME HELP SERVICE

Another most practical form of help for physically disabled people is the home help service. Most local authorities assess the need on physical limitations and will expect those financially able to pay for the service. This might require applicants to undergo a means test. This is another aspect covered under Section 2 of the *Chronically Sick and Disabled Persons Act*. Until all people entitled to this service claim it, the Department of Health and Social Security will never obtain a true picture of the overall need.

Most home helps are friendly, good-natured people who undertake the work for more than merely doing a job. They will undertake light housework, shopping and a little cooking. Again there is an overwhelming demand on the service and applicants cannot expect to have their help more than perhaps a few hours weekly. This varies however from area to area, and full details of the service can be obtained from local social services departments.

TELEPHONE

One of the facilities which local authorities are enabled to provide for severely disabled people under Section 2 of the *Chronically Sick and Disabled Persons Act* is a telephone. I feel that all people disabled to such a degree that they are prevented from leaving their property in an emergency, such as fire, should be connected to the outside world by telephone.

Unfortunately, most local authorities subject applicants for telephones to a means test and base requirement more on the period of time the disabled person is left on their own, rather than their physical limitations. What happens to a paraplegic at night may be overlooked. Only in bed is the true impact of not being able to walk fully realized; the wheelchair may roll away from the bed, the patient may be taken ill or the house catch fire – what then?

Installation and rental of a telephone is expensive and it is understandable that local authorities cannot provide all disabled people with telephones much as they might like to. All I can suggest to those who have been refused a telephone is to appeal. If you are still unsuccessful, think very hard about saving and paying for one yourselves. Remember: it is for your own safety.

SOCIAL SECURITY FINANCIAL BENEFITS

Entitlement to social security benefits varies considerably and depends largely upon individual domestic circumstances. Qualification for benefits such as sickness and invalidity allowance will depend upon the requisite number of weekly contributions having been paid to the National Insurance Scheme. The range of available benefits is truly remarkable and I feel the only satisfactory method of deciding entitlement is to obtain pamphlets on these benefits and to study the detailed rules and regulations governing availability.

The Department of Health and Social Security produce leaflets covering all benefits. Leaflet FBI (family benefits and pensions) is a small booklet which gives detailed information about most benefits available to various groups of people. Leaflet NI 146 is a catalogue of social security leaflets and leaflet NI 196 gives full details of social security benefit rates.

As social security rules and benefits change so frequently, patients are advised to obtain these three leaflets from their local social security office as a basic guide to further claims. Should difficulty be experienced in obtaining these or other leaflets, then write to the DHSS Leaflets Unit.

DHSS Leaflets Unit,
Block 4, Government Buildings,
Honeypot Lane,
Stanmore,
Middlesex, HA7 1AY.

Like many other forms of help available from the social services, financial benefits tend to be obscure. If experiencing difficulties with a claim applicants should seek the help and advice available from one of the many organizations I have listed. One such organization, Disability Alliance, has produced an excellent handbook on income benefits together with other useful information.

WHEELCHAIRS AND OTHER AIDS

WHEELCHAIRS

To the paraplegic the most useful single item of equipment supplied by the National Health Service is undoubtedly the wheelchair. These are issued to those who require them, free of charge, but they remain the property of the National Health Service. At the National Spinal Injuries Centre, Stoke Mandeville Hospital, the Everest & Jennings folding wheelchair has been found to be the most satisfactory chair for patients with spinal cord injuries, and the Department of Health and Social Security has recently agreed that this chair should be the type issued to continuing long-term physically disabled patients. They can be produced in many different sizes to accommodate individual needs. The more severely disabled with limited or no arm movements can be supplied with electrically-powered chairs produced by this company.

Regardless of the type of chair supplied, its value must be clearly understood, not in terms of cash, but as an aid to mobility. Without a wheelchair, the paraplegic will either be confined to bed, or at least an armchair inside the house. It can dramatically broaden the horizons of your life, and as all chairs are supplied on the understanding that users are responsible for their maintenance, cleaning and oiling – look after them well!

In most cases it is only possible to supply one wheelchair per person, but those supplied with electrically-powered chairs are also entitled to an ordinary chair to enable them to be taken out and to travel. Remember, **never** travel in a car without a wheelchair in case of a breakdown.

Patients in a financial position to purchase a second or third chair of their own (perhaps with a compensation claim) are well advised to do so. Thus if one chair breaks down, mobility is not impaired while repairs are being carried out. Wheelchairs are expensive, but when one considers emergencies such as fire there can be no price placed on mobility. Patients intending to purchase their own chair should obtain a certificate from their doctor stating that it is required on health grounds and the chair can then be bought free of V.A.T. (value added tax).

There are a number of different makes of wheelchairs besides the Everest & Jennings. Although this is the recommended chair, patients wishing to buy one of their own might like to try a different make. The Disabled Living Foundation stock most makes of wheelchairs and patients can go there and try them out.

Following discharge from hospital, the Department of Health and Social Security Artificial Limb and Appliance Centre (A.L.A.C.), in the paraplegic's home area, is the centre responsible for all problems and repairs to National Health Service wheelchairs. Their address can be found in the telephone directory under Health and Social Security, Department of. At regular intervals a technical officer from this centre will visit patients in their homes to inspect wheelchairs and arrange for any necessary repairs. Between his visits if minor repairs costing a maximum of £3.00 are required, they can be carried out under the orders of patients and receipts sent to the A.L.A.C. for reimbursement. More extensive repairs must be notified to the nearest A.L.A.C. and their official repairer will be responsible.

Wheelchairs should be inspected at regular monthly intervals. Nuts and bolts should be tightened and in particular the screws holding the backrest checked. The backrest material is inclined to tear by the top fixing screw, particularly when patients drape their arms over the backrest. During hot weather and in central heating conditions, the bearings soon dry out. These should be oiled or greased as recommended. Tyres should always be kept well inflated as soft tyres wear out more quickly and certainly make the task of pushing more difficult. Zimmer Orthopaedic supply a small tool kit and pump, together with maintenance instructions. These should be read carefully and the instructions followed.

Powered wheelchairs

The more severely disabled are, under certain circumstances, supplied with electrically driven wheelchairs for indoor use. These chairs are supplied on the same terms and conditions as ordinary chairs; namely that the user is responsible for maintenance, cleaning and oiling.

All recipients of powered wheelchairs from the Department of Health and Social Security are required to sign an undertaking that they will not use the chairs outdoors. The Department claims that none of the electrically driven wheelchairs issued are suitable for heavy outdoor use and that none match up to the specifications laid down in the regulations made under Section 20 of the *Chronically Sick and Disabled Persons Act*. Despite this Act and the written undertaking, Department officials agree that their chairs may be used outdoors with care 'within the curtilage of the residence'; and to save you looking that up in your dictionary it means a 'small courtyard attached to a dwelling house'.

Powered wheelchairs need not be registered or display number plates; they are also exempt from excise duty and from compulsory insurance requirements of the *Road Traffic Act 1960*. However users must consider suitable third-party insurance if the chair is to be used at regular times on pavements and crossing roads. RADAR issue an insurance policy at a reasonable premium.

The Everest & Jennings powered wheelchair is the make usually issued to the tetraplegic. These chairs can be fitted with several different types of controls, situated in any position to utilize any remaining movements the user may have. Chairs have been adapted to electromechanical, electropneumatic, breathing and even optical controls. The electromechanical control, where the control box can be mounted either for hand, foot, chin or head use appears to be the most suitable for the majority.

Many of the problems concerning failure of these chairs can be attributed to a poor understanding of basic maintenance. Chairs need to be inspected weekly and the nuts and bolts tightened. Particular attention should be paid to the Allen screws which hold pulleys on the motor drive shafts, as these sometimes wear loose. Care should be given to the vertical bolt that locates the motor mounting on the chair frame. This should be maintained in a 'pinched tight' position, thus ensuring that the spring or fibre locking nuts are secure. They should not be overtight, for the slight movement of the motor allows the drive pulleys to align when the drive belt is under tension. The drive belts require adjustment from time to time and should be regularly checked for wear. Adjustment is made by turning the bar nuts on the motor mountings, having first released the locking nuts. Drive belts that are adjusted incorrectly are often the cause of excessive wear and are responsible for the chair veering to one side when travelling.

BUYING A WHEELCHAIR When purchasing a wheelchair privately it may be possible to obtain hire purchase terms or a discount. Some companies which do arrange these facilities are listed below.

Biddle Engineering Co. Ltd., Hire purchase wheelchairs.
103, Stourbridge Road,
Halesowen,
West Midlands.
Telephone: ~~021–550 7426~~

Meyra Rehab (UK) Ltd., Discounts from $7\frac{1}{2}$ to $10\frac{1}{2}$
Unit 4, per cent off the retail
Copheap Lane, price of wheelchairs for
Warminster, Mobility Allowance
Wilts. beneficiaries.
Telephone: 215122

Newton Aids Ltd., No-deposit hire purchase
2a, Conway Street, on wheelchairs for Mobility
London W1. Allowance beneficiaries.
Telephone: 01–580 4218

Zimmer Orthopaedic Ltd., Extension of guarantee on
180, Brompton Road, electric wheelchairs for one
London SW3. year for Mobility Allowance
Telephone: 01–584 6416 beneficiaries.

BATTERIES The Everest & Jennings power drive chair is fitted with two 6 volt lead acid type batteries. These are filled with dilute sulphuric acid. If it is allowed to come in contact with the skin or clothing this will burn. Therefore **great care** *must be taken* when handling them. The acid level should be checked weekly. If it is found to be below the level of the plates, as seen through the filler caps, it should be topped up with *distilled water*. The plates should be covered by about 3mm (⅛in) of distilled water and no more. Overfilling will result in spillage when charging or handling. A proper battery filler spout can be obtained from most motor accessory shops. This fits to a bottle and will only allow 3mm of water to cover the plates. Distilled water can be purchased from most garages and accessory shops.

Where corrosion is found on terminals, the clamps should be removed and all traces thoroughly cleaned off. If this has been neglected for a long time, severe damage may have occurred to both clamps and battery posts and these could require replacing.

Difficulty in removing corroded terminals can be eased by washing them in a warm detergent solution. Before refitting the cleaned clamps, cover them and the battery posts with a light coating of lanolin ointment.

CHARGING BATTERIES New batteries should last three days or more without being re-charged if the chair is used under normal domestic circumstances. During the summer months and if the user lives in a hospital or institutional home, when the chair will be used more, charging will be required more frequently. Best results are obtained if the battery is allowed to run almost flat before charging. With the issued 5 amp charger, a charge for 12 hours from flat is all that is required. Overcharging will not extend the running time of the chair, it will only result in damage to the batteries. As batteries get older they will absorb less charge and will require more frequent topping-up with distilled water. Under normal conditions the average life span of batteries should be between 2 and 4 years, but this varies according to the make.

When the charger is connected to the chair, the needle of the ammeter should show a reading. If it remains at zero, there is a fault and the battery is not being charged. When this happens switch off the electricity supply immediately and check that the chair is switched to the top speed, and that the terminals of the batteries are clean and making good contact. Check that the fuses of the plug, chair and charger are not blown (chair and charger fuses might be of the make-and-break contact type; the red buttons then only require pushing in), and check that the mains output socket is working.

If all these points are satisfactory, then something more serious may be wrong requiring the attention of someone familiar with electrical circuits. Other faults with chairs might be connected with the motors or controls. These are complicated and should not be tampered with by an amateur. Contact your A.L.A.C.

As with the ordinary chairs, patients requiring electrically powered chairs and in a financial position to purchase a second chair of their own would be well advised to do so. There are many different makes to choose from; again a visit to the Disabled Living Foundation will prove worthwhile.

Besides the Everest & Jennings and many other makes of electrically driven wheelchairs available, there is a small range of a new concept in powered wheelchairs now being offered to disabled people to purchase for themselves. One such make is the 3- or 4-wheeled Batric chair. These are specially designed for outdoor use and are able to travel over quite rough ground. On the whole they are unsuitable for the tetraplegic; although I do know of one tetraplegic who has had a 3-wheel version specially adapted to his requirements and it would seem ideal. These vehicles are allowed on the roads without tax and insurance, because they qualify under the regulations of Section 20 of the *Chronically Sick and Disabled Persons Act*. This is providing that they are fitted with suitable brakes and that they do not travel faster than four miles an hour. It is not necessary for them to have lights, unless of course they are used after dark.

Advertisements for these and similar chairs are in the national press, or further information can be obtained from the Spinal Injuries Association. While still in hospital, patients requiring wheelchairs will have them ordered by the consultant in charge. After discharge, if a new chair is required, it is not necessary to contact a hospital consultant as general practitioners are now allowed to prescribe chairs.

WHEELCHAIR SEAT CUSHIONS   As an aid in the prevention of pressure sores, patients issued with wheelchairs are also supplied with a cushion on which to sit. These are produced in many different forms, and like wheelchairs, are supplied free of charge on the National Health Service but remain its property.

The majority of patients will be supplied with the standard latex foam sorbo-rubber cushion, measuring 45cm (18in) square by 10cm (4in) thick. The junior model is 40cm (16in) square by 10cm thick. Patients are advised not to sit on cushions of this type that are less than 10cm (4in) thick, unless they are under medical supervision. Most will find this type of cushion satisfactory for normal daily use.

With regular daily use the sorbo-rubber cushion soon deteriorates, the rubber becomes soft and eventually compresses to a solid state under very little weight, thus increasing the risks of pressure sores forming. To reduce this risk, cushions should be examined at regular weekly intervals and when they are found to be soft, they should be replaced. Under normal circumstances and providing care has been taken of cushions, they should last 6 months or more. Their life can be extended by preventing them getting wet and by removing them from wheelchairs overnight. This allows them to air, for they do tend to absorb moisture from the skin. When replacing a cushion in a wheelchair, turn it the other way about to ensure even wear.

Cushions should not be placed on hot pipes or close to open fires. Excessive heat will result in the rubber perishing. Minor wetness should be dried in sunlight, which also sterilizes the cushion, or by leaving it in a drying room or airing cupboard. Should the cushion become soiled through a bowel accident, it is best destroyed, for any attempt to wash it only rots the rubber.

New cushions are obtainable from appliance centres; there is often a considerable delay in their supply and they should therefore be ordered well in advance. In any case, a reserve cushion should always be available.

RIPPLE CUSHIONS   In recent years many companies throughout the world have been trying to produce a cushion that will reduce the risk of pressure sores forming on patients who are too disabled to lift themselves in the normal manner. One such company, Tally Surgical Instruments Limited, has produced the ripple-seat cushion. This cushion is constructed of a plastic material and works on the principle of inflating alternate tubular sections, so that for short periods of time, areas of the buttocks are suspended over the gaps produced.

Like all such aids they appear to work quite well with some patients, though others find them of no value. Because they are produced in a plastic material, they tend to make the skin sweat and the moisture is not absorbed; this increases the risk of pressure sores. Patients trying these cushions for the first time should take extra care and only use them for short periods at first, so that they can test their reaction. A 5cm (2in) thick sorbo-rubber cushion should be used under the ripple-cushion, for added protection and to raise the wheelchair user to the correct sitting position.

Ripple-cushions used with a wheelchair are powered by a small battery-operated pump which can be hung on the side of the chair. As the rechargeable batteries only last between 10 and 12 hours, users are advised to always have more than one ready-charged for use. There is a mains-operated pump like the one used with the ripple-mattress, that can be used with the ripple-cushion in a fixed position, such as an armchair.

Ripple-cushions are supplied through appliance centres on the recommendation of a hospital consultant or a general practitioner. Patients who find them satisfactory and can afford to purchase a second one for use in emergencies, are advised to do so. For like all mechanical aids they do break down from time to time.

Again I remind readers that the ripple-cushion, like all other cushions, will **not** prevent pressure sores. It is only an aid in their prevention but it may permit some patients to sit for longer periods without being lifted.

SHEEPSKINS Sheepskins have been used for a number of years in aiding the prevention of pressure sores. Basically all they do is absorb moisture from the skin, which otherwise promotes redness, chafing and ultimate cracking of the skin. They can be used on top of a 10cm (4in) sorbo-rubber cushion, or for lying on directly in bed.

Those who find them of benefit should remember that they require regular washing as instructed by the suppliers, otherwise they soon become hard and matted and can only result in causing additional pressure. Sheepskins are available through the National Health Service on a recommendation of a hospital consultant or general practitioner, and are supplied through an appliance centre.

GEL-CUSHIONS In the continued fight against pressure sores, many companies have been experimenting with, and producing, cushions filled with a synthetic gel-type material designed to represent body fat. One such cushion, the Spence-Gel cushion, produced by Everest & Jennings in Los Angeles, has been on trial at the National Spinal Injuries Centre. Results are similar to other aids; they suit some patients and not others. (I know of one person who claims to have sat for 18 hours without a lift and with no resultant damage. If that claim is true, to try and do this on a regular basis would, I feel certain, lead to problems in the future.)

No matter what kind of cushion is used, there will always be pressure problems caused by body weight. Some cushions may help reduce pressure to a minimum and when the individual is well padded with normal body fat and tissue, and has a good circulation, patients might be under the impression that the particular type of cushion they are using is working efficiently for them. In actual fact it is their own natural bodily functions doing the work under ideal conditions.

Gel-cushions are available on the recommendation of a hospital consultant and on prescription from the family doctor. They are available through local A.L.A.Cs.

OTHER TYPES OF CUSHIONS Where problems exist due to pressure and normal methods of prevention have failed, research, trial and close observation has to be undertaken to find a more suitable surface on which to sit. Medical advice should always be sought before trying different cushions. In many cases excessive pressure may be due to other causes than the cushion.

Often a combination of two cushions is of value, such as a 7·5cm (3in) and a 5cm (2in) sorbo-rubber put together making a 12·5cm (5in) thick cushion on which to sit. This certainly proved completely successful in my own case, when for several years I suffered constant effects of pressure over an old scar. I came to the conclusion that the quality of the 10cm (4in) cushion had deteriorated over the years making it less buoyant. Consequently the cushion compressed to a solid state under less weight. With the extra 2·5cm (1in) thickness afforded by using a 12·5cm (5in) thick cushion, there was a greater margin between the cushion becoming compressed to a solid and the period when it was still offering buoyance. I would recommend those with pressure problems to try this.

Cushions made of other synthetic materials, such as polystyrene beads, polystyrene foam rubber chips, together with numerous other combinations have not proved outstandingly successful, so if they are tried great caution should be observed.

Crutches, calipers and walking sticks

As part of medical rehabilitation, some patients, usually those with mid-thoracic and lower lesions, are taught to walk with the aid of calipers and crutches or walking sticks. The style of walking will vary depending on the level and extent of injury, but basically calipers are worn to lock the knees and to keep the legs straight. Walking is then achieved by using the upper limbs together with crutches or walking sticks which support and steady the trunk. This enables weight to be lifted off the legs either by tilting the pelvis and allowing alternate legs to move forward, or by swinging both legs through together.

Patients requiring calipers and crutches or walking sticks, will have them measured to fit whilst in hospital. Crutches and sticks are frequently of the telescopic adjustable type and are a standard issue. Calipers for paraplegics are expertly made. If difficulties are experienced, patients should try and have them adjusted by the original maker. If this is not possible, then ask your A.L.A.C. for help and advice. A.L.A.C. should be contacted for all problems connected with crutches and walking sticks.

10

Work and Play

EMPLOYMENT

Employment for both paraplegic and tetraplegic patients frequently requires further education and training in a new occupation. To help patients find suitable employment, a Disablement Resettlement Officer (D.R.O.) is available to give advice and possibly to arrange special training courses. In most cases the D.R.O. will visit patients before they are discharged from hospital, otherwise full details of this service can be obtained from local employment offices or job centres. Patients under 18 years of age should apply to the Youth Employment Centre.

Employment for paraplegics is obviously less difficult to obtain than it is for tetraplegics. However during a research project into employment for tetraplegics in which I was involved, we were delighted to discover the wide range of full and part-time occupations now being undertaken. The report on this research project entitled *Employment for Tetraplegics* is available from the National Fund for Research into Crippling Diseases, who were sponsors for the research.

Sir Ludwig Guttmann has been quoted as saying that his interpretation of fully rehabilitated paraplegics was to see them again as tax payers. How appropriate his words are when you consider the vast sums of tax payers' money spent on health care.

Naturally not every spinal injury patient will be capable of, or need to, return to employment. Much depends upon age, extent and location of injury, domestic circumstances and financial requirements. Nevertheless, employment is not just a means of earning money. Indeed quite often this is the last consideration. Employment provides a feeling of self-satisfaction and independence, of being able to compete with able-bodied members of society, of responsibility, pride and social status.

There is no reason why a paraplegic or tetraplegic should not marry, have or adopt children, take out insurance policies, obtain a mortgage and enter into hire purchase agreements. Most of these activities depend upon a stable, responsible background associated with a desire to seek employment.

Possum

Possum is the registered trade mark of Possum Controls Ltd., a company producing electronic and electro-mechanical equipment to give severely physically disabled persons a degree of control over their immediate environment.

The equipment, which is operated by depressing a simple microswitch or by sucking or puffing on a pneumatic tube, will switch on and off any number of electrical appliances that are connected to the control box such as a light, fan, fire alarm, television, radio, and tape recorder. Control of a telephone and dialling can also be provided. This equipment is available on the National Health Service and anybody severely physically disabled may apply for it to be installed in their home. Application should be made through a patient's own doctor to the Regional Medical Officer of the Regional Health Authority.

As well as the standard range of equipment that is available on the National Health Service, Possum Controls have produced controls for typewriters and other office machinery. Full details of their range of equipment can be obtained on request.

Recreation

Recreational activities, both within the home and hospital are vitally important to prevent boredom which frequently arises through restricted physical activities. During a patient's stay in hospital, the daily routine is often so demanding that little consideration is given to recreation after discharge. Most patients will admit that after discharge there is a period of inactivity when sheer boredom is experienced. This is due to the sudden switch from a very active and busy hospital routine filled with physiotherapy, swimming and occupational therapy, to days at home when all one has to consider is personal management.

Recreational activities are of course restricted to a certain degree. For example, it would prove difficult to rock-climb in a wheelchair! There are, however, many activities that can be carried out from a wheelchair with ease. Gardening, bird watching and photography are varied examples of outside activities which are popular among disabled people. Expeditions to concerts, theatres, and cinemas are possible; and active participation in amateur dramatics, a choir or playing an instrument can be enjoyed from a wheelchair. At home there are many sedentary pursuits to keep a patient occupied; from further education and study to carpentry and metal-work, from painting or craft work to chess or draughts. The possibilities are too many to list here but I include some appropriate addresses for further information.

Focus on Hobbies,
7, Rochester Row,
Northwood, Middlesex.
Telephone: Northwood 23013

Gardens for the Disabled Trust,
c/o Garden Club,
Lilac House,
Biddenden
Kent.

Photography for the Disabled,
190, Secrett House,
Ham Close,
Ham, Richmond,
Surrey.
Telephone: 01–948 2342

Radio Amateur Invalid and Bedfast Club,
Bristol Road,
Cambridge,
Glos. GL2 7DE.

Nottingham Handicraft Co.,	Suppliers of materials for
Melton Road,	handicrafts. (Basket and
West Bridgford,	leather-work, toys etc.)
Nottingham,	
NG2 6HD.	
Telephone: 0602 234251	

Sport

Sport, as an extension to the medical rehabilitation of paraplegic patients, was introduced by Sir Ludwig Guttmann during
his early pioneer days at Stoke Mandeville Hospital. His aim
was to use the medium of sport to strengthen non-paralysed
parts of the body and to create comradeship between disabled
people. In countless cases the sporting medium has played an
important role in social acceptance, adjustment and resettlement
of all kinds of disabled people.

Since those early pioneering days, sport for the disabled has
become recognized the whole world over as being a first class
method of keeping fit, promoting understanding between disabled people, and encouraging medical and paramedical staff
to improve standards of care for the disabled.

Today there is a world-wide paraplegic sports movement
which meets and partakes as part of the Olympic Games. There
is a wide range of sporting activities now undertaken by paraplegics including archery, table-tennis, basket-ball, fencing,
snooker and billiards, and swimming to mention just a few.
Sir Ludwig's recent textbook *Sport for the Disabled*, is an
invaluable guide for all connected with or interested in
sport.

There are many sports organizations, clubs and associations for paraplegics to join and seek further information. The following list indicates some of these associations:

The British Paraplegic Sports Society Ltd.,
Stoke Mandeville Sports Stadium for the Paralysed and other Disabled,
Harvey Road,
Aylesbury, Buckinghamshire.
Telephone: Aylesbury 84848

The British Sports Association for the Disabled,
Stoke Mandeville Sports Stadium for the Paralysed and other Disabled,
Harvey Road,
Aylesbury, Buckinghamshire.
Telephone: Aylesbury 84848

Riding for the Disabled Association,
National Agriculture Centre,
Kenilworth,
Warwickshire, CV8 2LY.
Telephone: Coventry 56107

Scottish Sports Association for the Disabled,
22, Charlotte Square,
Edinburgh,
EH2 4DF.
Telephone: 031–225 7282

Information on Water Sports,
The Sports Council,
70, Brompton Road,
London SW3.

National Anglers' Council Committee for Disabled Anglers,
5, Cowgate,
Peterborough PE1 1LR.
Telephone: 0733 54084

The Committee for the Promotion of Angling for the Disabled,
18–19, Claremont Crescent,
Edinburgh,
EH7 4QD.
Telephone: 031–556 3882

Great Britain Wheelchair Basketball League,
18, Wroxhall Drive,
Grantham,
Lincs. NG31 7EQ.

11
Transport

The ability and freedom to travel from A to B, either for business or pleasure, are equally important, but often very much more difficult for the disabled traveller than for the able-bodied person. In most cases the disabled are able to travel in exactly the same transport as that provided for the general public, although special thought may need to be given as to suitability, adaptations and modifications, time of journey and advance bookings.

Transport can be divided into two groups, public and privately owned. In relation to transport and travel for the paraplegic, private transport usually means a motor vehicle, whereas public transport includes travel by road, rail, air and to a lesser extent sea. This chapter relates to the more common methods of transport suitable to paraplegics.

PRIVATE TRANSPORT

The privately owned motor vehicle is undoubtably the most common and most satisfactory method of transport for the paraplegic. It is an almost, if not vital part of the basic necessary equipment required.

Until 1976 the Department of Health and Social Security issued specially constructed and adapted 3-wheeled invalid vehicles to disabled people who qualified under the regulations and who were able to drive them. Other special groups of people, such as disabled housewives with children of school age, were under certain circumstances issued with a 4-wheeled vehicle such as a Mini. Disabled drivers who wanted to purchase their own vehicles and have them suitably adapted, were able to claim a private car allowance and exemption from road tax. Disabled passengers who provided their own vehicle were also, under certain circumstances, exempt from paying road tax.

In an attempt to provide a wider range of help to all disabled people, the Department of Health and Social Security decided to stop any further issue of the invalid car (although those in service will be maintained until 1983) and to withdraw the car allowance. In place of these benefits, the Department has introduced a Mobility Allowance which is taxable and which will eventually be paid to all disabled people who qualify without age limit. The changes from the previous benefits are being introduced progressively between 1977 and 1978.

Certain ex-service personnel, war pensioners and those who became disabled whilst serving, are issued with 4-wheeled vehicles specially converted, regardless of whether they are able to drive. This scheme is unaffected.

Those people issued with 3-wheeled invalid vehicles can continue with the present arrangements, or if they wish, trade in the vehicle for the Mobility Allowance. Once this has been done, it cannot be reversed. Leaflet N1 211 obtainable from any social security office gives full details of the Mobility Allowance and includes the appropriate application form. *The Mobility Allowance (Vehicle Scheme Beneficiaries) Regulations, 1977*, SI No 1229, is available from H.M.S.O. price 15p.

How the recipient of the Mobility Allowance uses the cash benefit (paid at four-weekly intervals in arrears) in relation to transport, is entirely up to the individual concerned. It can be used to purchase a train or bus ticket, pay a taxi fare, or saved up to purchase an air or sea ticket to the other side of the world. Most people use the benefit towards the purchase and running expenses of a motor vehicle. As it can cost more to purchase, maintain and run a car, than to buy and maintain the average house, it is impossible to visualize how any element of the Mobility Allowance could be set aside for car purchase alone.

The Royal Association for Disability and Rehabilitation

(RADAR), is at present looking into the possibility of setting up an organization, similar to a finance company, for the purpose of supplying loans to the disabled to assist with car purchase. It is intended that such loans will be interest-free as RADAR will obtain its funds for lending from the Government.

In order to assist the disabled with the purchase of a suitable vehicle, several of the leading car manufacturers, including British Leyland, Vauxhall, Chrysler and Fiat, have agreed to offer a discount of 15 per cent on new vehicles to those in receipt of the Mobility Allowance. The discount is taken off the basic price only, and with car tax of 10 per cent and V.A.T. at 8 per cent added, the discount in relation to the total price is about 13 per cent. Vauxhall have offered this discount off all their vehicles, whilst British Leyland have excluded Rover, Jaguar and Daimler models.

The Ford Motor Company of Britain have gone one step further. They were first approached by the Thalidomide Trust, at St Neots, Cambridge, to assist in research aimed at providing thalidomide victims with vehicles which could be suitably adapted to individual needs, and as a result became more aware of the problems of disabled drivers generally. In conjunction with the Department of Health and Social Security; The Minister for the Disabled, Mr Alfred Morris; Dr Gerard Vaughan, F.R.C.P., M.P., Opposition Spokesman on Health; The Royal Association for Disability and Rehabilitation (then The Central Council for the Disabled), The Disabled Drivers' Motor Club; Feeny and Johnson Ltd.; and Reselco Invalid Carriages Ltd.; Ford have produced an Escort 1.3 Popular 2-door automatic with a six-part 'disability pack' which includes:

specially extended seat slide
heated rear window
remote-control driver's door mirror
laminated windscreen
hazard warning flashers
inertia reel seat belts

The Escort is being offered by Ford main dealers and the

current price which includes car tax and V.A.T. represents an overall discount of about 18 per cent. The car is available to disabled drivers and disabled learner drivers receiving the Mobility Allowance. The disabled driver will need to have suitable hand controls fitted, by either a specialist conversion firm, or by the Ford dealer.

Ford have also introduced a support programme for the Escort and the disabled driver and the two most important aspects are:

Special credit facilities through Ford Motor Credit Limited, allowing a deposit of 20 per cent, a repayment period of up to 48 months, and a flat rate of interest of $9\frac{1}{2}$ per cent.

All disabled drivers buying the Escort automatic will receive The Ford Priority Service Card, which assures them of breakdown assistance and priority repairs from all Ford dealers.

Initially the car will only be offered to disabled drivers, but the special credit facilities will be offered to the immediate families of MobilityAllowance recipients who do not themselves drive. Ford dealers will also give special consideration when their cars are being bought to transport disabled persons receiving the Mobility Allowance. If you have problems in obtaining these Ford facilities contact Ford Motor Company Ltd., Eagle Way, Brentwood Essex.

Any general queries about car transport should be referred to RADAR, 25, Mortimer Street, London W1N 8AB. RADAR organize a wide range of mobility concessions for the disabled.

(This information is correct at the time of press. It would be wiser if intending buyers checked these facts for themselves.)

HAND CONTROLS

Besides the cars mentioned, practically any type of car, be it sports or saloon, can be converted to hand controls to suit the paraplegic driver. Tetraplegic drivers will obviously have a more limited choice and in most cases will have to depend on vehicles fitted with automatic transmission. Tetraplegics with spinal cord lesions above cervical 6 will have great difficulties in driving vehicles fitted with internal combustion engines, a few have managed to drive electrically operated invalid vehicles, but generally speaking it is the level of injury which is the deciding factor as to whether a person can or cannot learn to drive.

There are many specialist companies producing hand controls of various types to suit different disabilities and types of motor vehicle. Some of the larger firms offer nation-wide and over-seas service. I suggest that potential drivers contact these firms for their advice before purchasing a particular car that requires conversion, and in the following lists I indicate some of these firms.

Automobile & Industrial Developments Limited, Queensdale Works, Queensthorpe Road, Sydenham, London, SE24 4PJ. *Telephone:* 01–698 3451

Specialists in conversions for all types of cars.

Brig-Ayd Controls, 1, Margery Lane, Tewin, Welwyn, Herts, AL6 OPJ. *Telephone:* 043–871 7419

Specialists in all types of conversions.

British School of Motoring, Disability Training School, 102, Sydney Street, Chelsea, London, SW3. *Telephone:* 01–352 1014

Assessment, driving tuition, and hand control conversions.

Cowal Medical Aids Limited, 32, New Pond Road, Holmer Green, Bucks, HP15 6SU. *Telephone:* Holmer Green 3065

Specialists in conversions for all vehicles.

P—E

Feeny & Johnson Limited,
Alperton Lane,
Wembley,
Middlesex, HAO 1JJ.
Telephone: 01–998 4458/9

Provide a nation and world-wide service. Write to head office for full details of service and controls.

Midland Cylinder Rebores Limited,
Torrington Avenue,
Coventry.
Telephone: Coventry 462424

Specialists in all types of conversions.

Reselco Invalid Carriages Limited,
262–264, King Street,
Hammersmith,
London, W6.
Telephone: 01–748 5053/4

Specialists in conversions for all types of cars.

Wood's Disabled Drivers Centre,
626, Keppochhill Road,
Glasgow, Scotland.
Telephone: 041–332 7467

Specialists in all types of conversions.

Car hire

Some car hire firms arrange special discounts for Mobility Allowance beneficiaries and N.H.S. vehicle service. Kenning Car Hire charge $17\frac{1}{2}$ per cent less than their regular rates and Chrysler also give a discount.

Motoring organizations

Besides the Automobile Association and the Royal Automobile Club, there are other associations and clubs that cater exclusively for the disabled driver and passenger, and provide an excellent source of information on every aspect of disabled motoring. Membership entitles drivers to many concessions such as free travel on certain car ferries to the Continent, Channel Islands, Isle of Wight and Ireland. Full details of membership and benefits are obtainable by writing to the following addresses:

The Disabled Drivers' Association,
Ashwellthorpe,
Norwich, NR16 1EX.
Telephone: Fundenhall 499

Produce the national
magazine *The Magic Carpet*. Free to members – 4
issues yearly. Also owns
Ashwellthorpe Holiday
Hotel.

Disabled Drivers' Motor Club
Limited,
39, Templewood,
Ealing,
London, W13 8DU.
Telephone: 01–998 1226

Publish *The Disabled
Driver* every other month.
A newspaper full of information on all aspects of
motoring.

Disabled Motorists' Federation,
15, Rookery Road, Tilston
Malpas,
Cheshire,
Telephone: Tilston 373

All information about
disabled driving

DISABLED PASSENGERS

The choice of vehicle becomes even more important when the
disabled person is a passenger because of severe disability. The
disabled passenger is also entitled to the Mobility Allowance,
and this can be used to purchase and convert a vehicle if so required. Most disabled passengers manage to travel quite successfully in an ordinary car driven by a friend or relative. Much
depends on the attendant's ability to transfer the disabled person from wheelchair to car. This can be achieved by using a
sliding board, or by standing out of the chair into the car. The
need for adequate safety straps in addition to the normal seat
belts cannot be stressed enough for the more severely disabled
person, who might not be able to hold on.

An alternative method of transferring the more severely disabled person is with a hoist. Hoists seem to be used less frequently
as those experiencing difficulties transferring are turning towards

vehicles that can carry the disabled person sitting in the wheel-chair. Suitable for this purpose include:

Mini-Van Conversion,
Modern Vehicle Construction Ltd.,
Darwin Close, Off Commercial Road,
Reading, Berks.

Has a raised roof, double doors and a portable ramp.

Mini-Van Conversion,
Roots Maidstone Ltd.,
Mill Street,
Maidstone, Kent, ME15 6YD.

Has raised roof, horse-box type tail-gate.

DBS Garages (Cranleigh) Ltd.,
High Street,
Cranleigh,
Surrey, GU6 8AG.

Conversion of the Renault 4 high roof van. Has portable ramps.

Further details on these and other similar conversions can be obtained by writing to the firms listed or by contacting one of the disabled motorists' organizations.

Other organizations concerned with transport problems

All disabled people, whether drivers or passengers, will from time to time find difficulties regarding their entitlements, the law, or simply technical matters connected with choice of vehicles and their conversion. There exists an organization fully equipped to give advice on all these matters, so if in doubt write to:

The Joint Committee on Mobility for the Disabled,
Wanborough Manor,
Wanborough,
Guildford, Surrey, GU3 2JR.
Telephone: Guildford 810484

If you have problems with insurance, write to:

Disabled Drivers' Insurance Bureau,
292, Hale Lane,
Edgware,
Middlesex HA8 8NO
Telephone: 01–958 3135

Car badge scheme

The car badge scheme for disabled drivers and passengers was
introduced in December 1971 and entitles people with defects of
the spine or central nervous system, or those dependent on the
use of wheelchairs, to certain parking concessions. These include
indefinite periods of free parking at meters and in areas where
time limits apply. Details of the scheme can be found through
application to local social services departments. A charge of
£1.00 for the orange badge may be made. The scheme is valid
throughout England, Scotland and Wales except for the following areas of central London: the City of London, the City of
Westminster, the London Borough of Camden south of and
including Euston Road, and the Royal Borough of Kensington
and Chelsea. If you live in one of these areas, you can apply for
an orange badge for use elsewhere, as well as the special local
badge. Local badges are only valid in the borough where they
are issued.

PUBLIC TRANSPORT

BRITISH RAIL

Travel by British Rail for the wheelchair user can present problems, and British Rail recommend all severely disabled people
to advise them well in advance of any intended journey. When
regular journeys are made, staff employed at the stations concerned soon learn of the disabled person's needs and are most
helpful in every way possible. For the occasional journey, it is

reasonable to ask that station staff are informed when a disabled person will be travelling on a certain train. British Rail have issued the following instructions to disabled travellers: 'Please write to the Area Manager at the departure station giving the following information:

1. Date and time of intended journey.
2. To where you are travelling and list of stations where changes have to be made.
3. Whether you are totally dependent on your wheelchair.
4. Whether you will be alone or with a travelling companion.
5. Whether you wish to travel in the guard's van or whether you are able to transfer out of your wheelchair and sit in an ordinary passenger seat. (To do this it might be necessary to be transported in a special narrow transit chair along train corridors.)'

Fare concessions

Under certain circumstances British Rail allow reductions in the fare normally charged. Those travellers who elect to travel in the guard's van, either because they cannot transfer or because they do not wish to, are charged half the normal second class single fare for each journey made and this also applies to one travelling companion. Written permission is required to do this and there are two different application forms and permits, one for regular travellers (form BR 25559/1), the other for single journeys (form BR 25559/2). They enable any passenger, disabled or not, to travel in non-passenger vehicles.

Passengers who prefer to travel in an ordinary passenger seat have to pay the normal fare. The wheelchair has then to be carried in the guard's van at no charge providing it folds and weighs less than 27kg (60lbs). If it is unable to fold and weighs more than the permitted limit, then a charge at the normal rate for accompanied items will be made.

Access to trains

The modern Inter-City coaches are constructed with wider doors than the older coaches, corridors are also wider. If the wheelchair is no wider than 65cm (25½in), then the wheelchair can be lifted on board and wheeled to a suitable seat where the occupant has then to transfer and stow the wheelchair in the guard's van. British Rail's Mark III first class coaches are constructed with a seat and table that can be removed and the traveller can remain sitting in the wheelchair, providing it is not more than 63cm (24½in) wide. Although these are first class coaches, British Rail charge a second class fare for the wheelchair user and for his companion.

The majority of mainline stations are accessible to wheelchairs, but difficulty may be experienced in getting from platform to platform and routes used for baggage and mail may have to be taken. Toilets are usually accessible, but not all are 'unisex'. Toilets on trains however are all unsuitable for wheelchair users and in circumstances where a journey cannot be made without toilet facilities, then it might be necessary to reserve a whole compartment. This can be done at a charge of 6 adult fares. However the older coaches with individual compartments are slowly being replaced with 'open-plan' style coaches, so this service will eventually be withdrawn.

Other services which might be of benefit to the disabled traveller include Motorail and Sleeper services; complete information on these and other services can be obtained from most British Rail stations or by purchasing a copy of *A Guide to British Rail – a handbook for the Disabled Person* available from the Royal Association for Disability and Rehabilitation (RADAR). The Joint Committee on Mobility for the Disabled also produce a leaflet called *British Rail and Disabled Travellers*.

TRAVEL BY BUS

Except in the case of patients with very incomplete lesions who are able to walk fairly well, travel by public bus service is, for obvious reasons, quite unsuitable for the wheelchair user. (I do know of one paraplegic woman who travels regularly on buses with her able-bodied husband. He carries her to a seat, then folds and stores her wheelchair in the luggage compartment.) In theory this is possible, but in practice buses are not provided with much luggage space and the conductor has the right to refuse entry to any passenger.

There are several privately owned buses belonging to hospitals, charities or disabled associations, which have been specially adapted to carry wheelchairs. This usually requires the removal of the ordinary seats, the addition of wheelchair locking devices and special safety straps together with either an electric or hydraulic operated tail-lift.

TRAVEL BY TAXI

Travel by taxi is perfectly possible and is frequently used by many wheelchair users. It would be wise to seek a regular taxi firm or driver if many journeys are anticipated, as they will then learn some of the problems of wheelchair users. Tetraplegics who are unable to transfer themselves, cannot expect the taxi driver to be willing to lift them in and out of their wheelchairs. Previous arrangements should always be made under these circumstances and an assistant taken. Most taxi drivers are very generous and willing to lift/help disabled people in and out if necessary.

TRAVEL BY AIR

Paraplegics who anticipate travelling by air are advised to write to the Airline Users Committee, who produce a booklet called *Care In The Air*. This booklet outlines all the problems and difficulties likely to be experienced.

The larger airports, such as Heathrow, produce their own booklets regarding who looks after disabled travellers. Your local travel agent is the best person to give advice.

From a medical point of view, under normal circumstances paralysis does not prevent air travel, although a check-up before a journey is always a wise precaution. The more severely disabled, who are unable to totally care for themselves, will in most circumstances require an assistant to travel with them.

Airline Users Committee,   Further information about
Space House,   air travel.
43–59, Kingsway,
London, WC2B 6TE.

TRAVEL BY SEA

Many large shipping companies cater for wheelchair passengers and your local travel agent is the best person to turn to for initial information. (See Appendix.)

Glossary

automatic bladder: this is one which will empty as the result of stimulation of its reflex action, i.e. tapping.

autonomic dysreflexia: this is the excessive rise in blood pressure, resulting in a thumping headache, due to stimulation of bladder, bowel or uterus. It is of a reflex nature, experienced mainly by cervical and high thoracic lesions.

autonomous bladder: this is one with no reflex action but which can be emptied by supra-pubic manual pressure at regular intervals.

catheter: this is a rubber or plastic tube to allow the passage of fluids, particularly of the bladder.

cauda equina: this is literally the horse's tail, the bundle of sacral and lumbar nerves at the base of the spinal column.

claustrophobia: this is fear of closed-in spaces.

contracture: this is permanent shortening of the tendon or muscle fibres, due to wrong positioning.

electrotherapy: this is treatment by electrical currents, e.g. faradism, galvanism, short-wave diathermy.

Guttmann's sign: this is the blockage of nasal air passages following a cervical spinal cord injury – caused through interruption of sympathetic nervous system. The blockage in the nasal air passage will impede respiration.

hydrotherapy: this is treatment by water, e.g. exercising in heated pools.

osteomyelitis: this is inflammation of the marrow of the bone.

osteoporosis: this is thinning of the bones due to the reabsorption of calcium; frequently occurs with disuse of limbs.

paramedical: this is a term used to describe staff other than nursing and medical, who are professionally qualified, e.g. physiotherapists, chiropodists, occupational and speech therapists.

rehabilitation: this is the restoration of a person to as near a normal condition as is possible, following injury or illness.

spasms: these are involuntary movements of muscles and may be convulsive in nature.

symphysis pubis: this is the bony prominence at the front of the pelvis where the pubic bones join.

trauma: this is a condition of the body produced by injury or external violence.

traumatic: relating to trauma, particularly of injury.

Appendix of Helpful Organizations

The whole subject of aids and equipment to help disabled people gain greater independence is indeed big business. Aids vary from the simple walking stick to extremely expensive electronic equipment for the more severely disabled commercially referred to as Possum.

Being suddenly confronted with physical disability, either as a patient, friend or relative, there is a natural desire to look around for aids and gadgets that might widen the disabled person's horizon. Long before the stage of getting out of bed into a wheelchair is reached, many families consider buying this and that, changing their cars, altering their houses, believing their disabled relative will need all these things for survival. I can even recall one family who went to the length of having electrically-operated doors fitted to their house within 10 weeks of their 20 year old son becoming paraplegic. All they really required was to have the doors made wider and the latch and lock lowered. That particular family could have saved themselves a lot of money if only they had waited until their son had got up in his wheelchair and discovered what he could or could not do.

This is precisely the key to the whole problem and much private and Health Service money could be saved in not ordering aids and equipment that are totally unnecessary and never used.

Apart from making basic house alterations and providing essential aids such as a suitable bed, my advice is to postpone buying extra aids and equipment until after the disabled person has been discharged and has had time to explore his limitations. Often families would benefit by seeking help and advice from someone experienced in assessing the capabilities of disabled people. One such person, Roger Jefcoate, the only independent consultant adviser for aids and equipment in the whole country, has had many years of experience in assessing and offering practical advice and assistance on specific needs to handicapped people from all walks in life.

Mr. Roger Jefcoate,
Willowbrook,
Swanbourne Road,
Mursley, Milton Keynes,
Bucks. MK17 OJA.
Telephone: Mursley 533

AIDS AND EQUIPMENT

Biological Engineering Society,
Handicap Advisory and Rehabilitation Group,
c/o Keith Copeland,
Dept. of Biophysics,
University College,
Gower Street,
London WC1.
Telephone: 01–387 7050 – ext. 288

Specialist advice – unusual equipment

Disabled Living Centre,
84, Suffolk Street,
Birmingham 1.
Telephone: 021–643 0980

Exhibition of aids and equipment.

Disabled Living Foundation,
346, Kensington High Street,
London W14.
Telephone: 01–602 2491

Provides a comprehensive display of aids and equipment that can be tried. It also provides an excellent information centre.

Dudley Controls Ltd.,   Makers of electronic
34, High Street,   controls for wheel-
Aylesbury,   chairs.
Buckinghamshire.
Telephone: Aylesbury 5231

Egerton Hospital Equipment Ltd.,   Makers of electric and
Tower Hill,   other turning beds.
Horsham, Surrey.
Telephone: Horsham 3800

G.U. Manufacturing Co. Ltd.,   Suppliers of rubber
28a, Devonshire Street,   urinals – colloquially
London W1.   known as 'kippers'.

H. & C. Lifts,   Makers of lifts.
159, St. John Street,
London EC1V 4JQ.

Interlock Systems for the Disabled, Produce many simple
The Spastics Society,   electrical and
Sherrards Industrial Centre,   electronic aids at
Digswell Hill,   reasonable prices.
Old Welwyn, Herts.

Maling Rehabilitation   Electronic environ-
Systems Ltd.,   mental control
St. Andrews Way,   systems. Advisory
Industrial Estate,   service.
Bicester Road,
Aylesbury, Buckinghamshire.
Telephone: Aylesbury 86521

Merseyside Aids Centre,   Exhibition of aids and
Youens Way,   equipment.
East Prescot Road,
Liverpool L14 2EP.

Newcastle Aids Centre, Mea House, Ellison Place, Newcastle-upon-Tyne. *Telephone:* 0632–23617	Exhibition of aids and equipment.
Possum Research Foundation, *also* Possum Controls Ltd., 63, Mandeville Road, Aylesbury, Buckinghamshire. *Telephone:* Aylesbury 81591	Makers of POSM electronic equipment.
The Royal Association for Disability and Rehabilitation (RADAR), 25 Mortimer Street, London W1N 8AB. *Telephone:* 01–637 5400	Has a travelling exhibition of aids.
Spastics Society, 12, Park Crescent, London W1N 4EQ. *Telephone:* 01–636 5020	Has mobile exhibition.
Tally Surgical Instruments Ltd., 47, Theobald Street, Boreham Wood, Herts. *Telephone:* 01–953 7171	Makers of ripple cushions and mattresses.
Terry Personal Lifts, Knutsford, Cheshire. *Telephone:* Knutsford 3211	Makers of interfloor lifts.
Vessa Ltd., Queen Mary's Hospital, Roehampton, London S.W.15. *Telephone:* 01–788 4422	Makers of wheelchairs.

Vitafoam Ltd., Don Mill, Middleton, Manchester 4.	Makers of sorbo- rubber packs.
Wessex Medical Equipment Co., The Hundred, Romsey, Hampshire. *Telephone:* 0794–518246	Makers of electric hoists, lifts and other medical equipment including beds.
Zimmer Orthopaedic Ltd., Bridgend, Glamorgan, Wales.	Makers of wheelchairs and other equipment.

BOOKS AND PUBLICATIONS

B. Fallon, *so you're paralysed*	Published by the Spinal Injuries Association.
Dr. Wendy Greengross, *Entitled to Love*	Most explicit book on the sexual aspects of disability. Published by Malaby Press, London, in association with the National Fund for Research into Crippling Diseases, 1, Springfield Road, Horsham, Sussex.
Sir Ludwig Guttmann, *Sport for the Disabled*	Published by H. M. & M. Publishers, Aylesbury.

Joanna Johnson,
Working at Home

Information on home employment. Penguin edition.

Dr. J. J. Walsh,
Understanding Paraplegia

Published by Tavistock.

AA Guide for the Disabled,
AA Hotel Services Dept.,
P.O. Box 52,
Basingstoke,
Hants.

General useful information relating to suitable accommodation and travelling.

ABC of Services and Information,
Disablement Income Group, (DIG)
28, Commercial Street,
London E1.

The Cord magazine,
Editor, Miss J. Scrutton,
Stoke Mandeville Sports Stadium,
Harvey Road,
Aylesbury, Bucks.

General useful information relating to paraplegia – facts and information on experiences.

Possibility magazine,
Secretary, Mr. R. A. Bowell,
'Copper Beech,'
Parry's Close,
Stoke Bishop,
Bristol, BS9 1AW.

Magazine of the Possum Users' Association. General information.

CAR CONVERSIONS

Automobile & Industrial
Developments Limited,
Queensdale Works,
Queensthorpe Road,
Sydenham, London SE24 4PJ.
Telephone: 01–698 3451

Specialists in
conversions for all
types of cars.

Brig-Ayd Controls,
1, Margery Lane,
Tewin, Welwyn,
Herts, AL6 OPJ.

Specialists in all types
of conversions.

Cowal Medical Aids Ltd.,
32, New Pond Road,
Holmer Green,
Bucks, HP15 6SU.
Telephone: Holmer Green 3065

Specialists in
conversions for all
vehicles.

DBS Garages (Cranleigh) Ltd.,
High Street,
Cranleigh,
Surrey, GU6 8AG.

Conversion of the
Renault 4 high roof
van. Has portable
ramps.

Feeny & Johnson Ltd.,
Alperton Lane,
Wembley,
Middlesex, HAO 1JJ.
Telephone: 01–998 4458/9

Provide a nation and
worldwide service.
Write to head office
for full details of
service and controls.

Midland Cylinder Rebores Ltd.,
Torrington Avenue,
Coventry.
Telephone: Coventry 462424

Specialists in all types
of conversions.

Mini-Van Conversion, Modern Vehicle Construction Ltd., Darwin Close, off Commercial Road, Reading, Berks.	Has a raised roof, double doors and a portable ramp.
Mini-Van Conversion, Roots Maidstone Ltd., Mill Street, Maidstone, Kent, ME15 6YD.	Has raised roof, horse-box type tail-gate.
Reselco Invalid Carriages Ltd., 262–264 King Street, Hammersmith, London, W6. *Telephone:* 01–748 5053/4	Specialists in conversions for all types of cars.
Wood's Disabled Drivers' Centre, 626, Keppochhill Road, Glasgow, Scotland. *Telephone:* 041–332 7467	Specialists in all types of conversions.

COUNSELLING

Throughout the lives of most people there are stress periods when, for various reasons, it is necessary to seek help and advice or just to talk to an outsider about certain problems.

The Spinal Injuries Association recognizes the ever-demanding need for a proper counselling service specifically designed to fit the special needs of paraplegics. Until such a service is established, there are various organizations in existence that a paraplegic can turn to for help and advice during periods of stress. These organizations have branches all over the country that can be found in the telephone directory, or by contacting the head offices:

Alcoholics Anonymous,
P.O. Box 514,
11, Redcliffe Gardens,
London S.W.10.
Telephone: 01–351 3344

For drinking
problems.

British Association for
Counselling,
26, Bedford Square,
London WC1B 3HU.
Telephone: 01–636 4066

All information
regarding every aspect
of counselling.

National Marriage Guidance
Council,
Herbert Grey College,
Little Church St.,
Rugby,
Warwickshire.
Telephone: Rugby 73241

Marital problems –
counselling.

The Samaritans,
39, Walbrook,
London E.C.4.
In local telephone directory under
SAMARITANS.

Depression –
suicide.

Scottish Marriage Guidance
Council,
58, Palmerston Place,
Edinburgh, EH12 5AZ.

Marital problems –
counselling.

Sexual Problems of the Disabled
(SPOD)
49 Victoria Street,
London SW1.
Telephone: 01–222 6067

Sexual problems of all
kinds, also
information.

ADOPTION

Adoption Resource Exchange,
40, Brunswick Square,
London WC1.
Telephone: 01–837 0496

Adoption.

British Adoption & Fostering
Agencies,
4, Southampton Row,
London WC1B 4AA.
Telephone: 01–242 8951

Provides lists of
agencies and advice.

National Adoption Society,
47a, Manchester Street,
Nr. Baker Street,
London W1.
Telephone: 01–935 7211

Adoption.

National Children Adoption
Association,
71, Knightsbridge,
London SW1.
Telephone: 01–235 6436

Standing Conference of Societies
Registered for Adoption,
Gort Lodge,
Petersham,
Surrey.
Telephone: 01–940 2646

Lists of registered
adoption societies.

ARTIFICIAL INSEMINATION

Artificial insemination either by donor or by husband, is now
available on the National Health Service. People considering
taking advantage of this facility should speak with their family
doctor in the first instance, or write to The Medical Director,

The Margaret Pyke Centre, 27–35, Mortimer Street, London, W1A 4QW. This centre is one of several in the country and they can provide basic information on request. There might however be a centre nearer your home, so speak with your family doctor first.

EDUCATION

The Advisory Centre for Education (ACE), 32, Trumpington Street, Cambridge.

Advice on all educational matters.

Association for Special Education, 19, Hamilton Road, Wallasey, Cheshire L45 9VE. *Telephone:* 051–522 3451

For children.

Council for Accreditation of Correspondence Colleges, 27, Marylebone Road, London NW1. *Telephone:* 01–935 5391

Has lists and information relating to courses.

National Institute of Adult Education, 35, Queen Anne Street, London W1.

Full information on courses and classes through local educational departments.

Open University Degree Courses, Open University, P.O. Box 48, Bletchley, Buckinghamshire.

Further degree standard education. A most helpful and progressive body in meeting educational requirements of the disabled.

The Royal Association for Disability and Rehabilitation (RADAR), 25, Mortimer Street, London W1N 8AB. *Telephone:* 01–637 5400 — Information and advice on education problems.

FINANCE

The AIDIS Trust, Sutton Waldron, Blandford, Dorset. — Financial support for the purchase of aids and equipment.

Birmingham Settlement Money Advice Centre, 318, Summer Lane, Birmingham B19 3RL. *Telephone:* 021–359 3562 — Debt counselling agency.

Child Poverty Action Group, 1, Macklin Street, London WC2. — Financial advice and information.

Citizen's Advice Bureaux 26, Bedford Square, London WC1B 3HU *Telephone:* 01–636 4066 Also local offices. — Advice on hire purchase, mortgages, tax, insurance etc.

Citizen's Rights Office, 1, Macklin Street, Drury Lane, London WC2B 5NH. — Will represent people at tribunals, advice over means-tests, supplementary benefits, all at no cost.

Claimants' Union, The Albany, Creek Road, London SE8. *Telephone:* 01–612 1047 — Self-help groups, assist in benefit claims and appeals.

Disability Alliance,
96, Portland Place,
London W.1.
Telephone: 01–794 1536

Advice and
information on
social security
benefits.

Disablement Incomes Group
(DIG), Attlee House,
Toynbee Hall,
28, Commercial Street,
London E1 6LR.
Telephone: 01–247 6877

Pressure group –
fights for better
economic and social
position for all disabled.
Advice on social
security benefits.

The Family Fund, Joseph Rowntree
Memorial Trust,
P.O. Box 50,
York YO3 6RB.

Financial help to
families with severely
handicapped children
from birth.

The Royal Association for Disability
and Rehabilitation (RADAR),
25, Mortimer Street,
London W1N 8AB.
Telephone: 01–637 5400

Produce leaflets on
such matters as income
tax, rate rebates.

GENERAL WELFARE

Association of Disabled Professionals,
c/o Mrs P. Marchant,
The Stables,
73, Pound Road,
Banstead, Surrey.

British Red Cross Society,
9, Grosvenor Crescent,
London SW1X 7EJ.
Telephone: 01–235 5454

Greater London Association
for the Disabled,
1, Thorpe Close,
London W10 5XL.
Telephone: 01–960 5799

Patients' Association,   Information and public
335, Grays Inn Road,   relations.
London WC1X 8PX.
Telephone: 01–837 7241

PHAB (Physically Handicapped and   Organization
Able Bodied) Clubs,   providing social
42, Devonshire Street,   meetings, sport,
London W1N 1LN.   education, mainly for
Telephone: 01–637 7475   the young disabled.

Queen Elizabeth's Foundation   General welfare,
for the Disabled,   education, rehabil-
Leatherhead,   itation, recreation,
Surrey, KT22 OBN.   holidays.
Telephone: Oxshott 2204

The Royal Association for   General information
Disability and Rehabilitation   and advice on
(RADAR),   education, employ-
25, Mortimer Street,   ment, fund raising etc.
London W1N 8AB.
Telephone: 01–637 5400

Scottish Information Service   General information.
for the Disabled,
18, Claremount Crescent,
Edinburgh,
Scotland EH7 4QD.
Telephone: 031–556 3882

Scottish Paraplegic Association,
3, Cargill Terrace,
Edinburgh
Scotland EH5 3ND.
Telephone: 031–522 8459

Spinal Injuries
Association of
Scotland. General
information.

Spinal Injuries Association,
126, Albert Street,
London NW1 7NE.
Telephone: 01–267 6111

All information
relating to
paraplegia. This is an
association for all
connected with spinal
injuries.

HOLIDAYS AND TRAVEL

Across Trust,
c/o Trade and Technical Press Ltd.,
Crown House,
Morden, Surrey.

Have Coach
ambulances to take
disabled people on
holiday.

Airline Users Committee,
Space House,
43–59, Kingsway,
London WC2B 6TE.

Further information
about air travel.

British Airports Authority,
Press and Public Relations,
Queen's Building,
Heathrow Airport, London,
Hounslow, Middlesex.

Provide a free booklet
giving details about
facilities for disabled
people at Heathrow
(also available from
the Disabled Living
Foundation).

Cunard Steamship Company Ltd.,
Passenger Reservations,
15, Regent Street,
London SW1 4LY.
Telephone: 01–930 7890

Information on
cruising.

Disabled Campers Club,
28, Coote Road,
Bexleyheath,
Kent DA7 4PR.
Telephone: 01–303 0753

Disabled Drivers' Association,
Ashwellthorpe,
Norwich, NR16 1EX.
Telephone: Fundenhall 449

Own Ashwellthorpe
Holiday Hotel.
Produce the national
magazine *The Magic
Carpet*, free to
members – 4 issues
a year.

Disabled Drivers' Motor Club,
39, Templewood,
Ealing,
London W13 8DU

Special concessions
with car ferry crossings
to the Continent, Isle
of Wight and
Channel Islands.

P and O Lines,
P and O Buildings,
Leadenhall Street,
London EC3.

Information on
cruising.

The Royal Association for Disability
and Rehabilitation (RADAR),
25, Mortimer Street,
London W1N 8AB.
Telephone: 01–637 5400

Provide a guide book
called *Holidays for the
Disabled* which lists
all suitable accom-
modation. They also
produce *Access to
Public Conveniences*.

Scottish Tourist Board,
23, Ravelston Terrace,
Edinburgh EH4 3EU.

Publish information
sheet for the disabled.

Wales Tourist Board,   Publish disabled
Welcome House,   visitors' guide to
High Street,   Wales.
Llandaff,
Cardiff CF5 272.

HOMES AND RESIDENTIAL
ACCOMMODATION

British Home and Hospital for Incurables,
Crown Lane,
Streatham,
London SW16 3JB.

Cheshire Foundation Homes for the
Sick,
7, Market Mews,
London W1Y 8HP.
Telephone: 01–499 2665

Duchess of Gloucester House,   Hostel for working
Ridgeway Road,   paraplegics.
Isleworth,
Middlesex.

Elizabeth Fitzroy Homes for the
Handicapped,
The Coach House,
Whitegates,
Liss, Hampshire.
Telephone: Liss 3577

John Groom's Association for the
Disabled,
10, Gloucester Drive,
London N4.
Telephone: 01–802 7272

Kytes Estate, Garston, Watford, Herts.	Bungalow settlement for paraplegics.
Lyme Green Settlement, Macclesfield, Cheshire.	Bungalow and single accommodation for paraplegics.
Papworth and Enham Village Settlement, The White House, Enham, Andover, Hampshire.	Provide accommo- dation and employ- ment where one or both partners is disabled.
Shaftesbury Society, 112, Regency Street, London SW1P 4AX.	Maintains special homes for young physically disabled men.
Star and Garter Home, Richmond Hill, Richmond, Surrey.	
Thistle Foundation, 22, Charlotte Street, Edinburgh EH2 4DF. *Telephone:* 031–225 7782	

MISCELLANEOUS INFORMATION

Carr's Rehabilitation Employment Advisory Service, 48, William IV Street, London WC2. *Telephone:* 01–836 5506	A private company that specializes in obtaining employment for disabled people.

Centre on Environment for the Handicapped, 126, Albert Street, Camden, London NW1 7NE. *Telephone:* 01–267 6111	Advice and guidance about house design.
Disabled Drivers' Insurance Bureau, 292, Hale Lane, Edgware, Middlesex. HA8 8NB *Telephone:* 01–958 3135	Advice about insurance.
The Joint Committee on Mobility for the Disabled, Wanborough Manor, Wanborough, Guildford, Surrey, GU3 2JR. *Telephone:* Guildford 810484	Advice and information about transport problems.
Legal Aid, New Legal Aid, P.O. Box 9, Nottingham NG1 6DS	Advice and information regarding legal aid.
The National Federation of Housing Associations, 86, Strand, London WC2R OEG. *Telephone:* 01–836 2741	Guide to all housing associations.

Rates relief. Most physically disabled people are entitled to rates relief, at least on their garage. Apply to your local valuation officer for further details.

Voting. Physically disabled people are entitled to postal voting, apply to your local electoral registrar for details.

RESEARCH AND DEVELOPMENT

Action Research for the Crippled
Child, Vincent House,
1, Springfield Road, Horsham,
W. Sussex, RH12 2PN.
Telephone: Horsham 64101

National Fund for Research into
Crippling Diseases, Vincent House,
1, Springfield Road, Horsham,
W. Sussex, RH12 2PN.
Telephone: Horsham 64101

REMAP c/o British Council for Rehabilitation of the Disabled, Thames House North, Millbank, London, SW1P 4QG.	Panels of engineers – give advice on adaptations and design new devices.

SPECIALIZED SPINAL INJURY UNITS

Aylesbury	The National Spinal Injuries Centre, Stoke Mandeville Hospital, Aylesbury, Bucks. *Telephone:* Aylesbury 84111
Belfast	Musgrove Park Hospital, Balmoral, Belfast BT9 7JB. *Telephone:* Belfast 66951

Cardiff	The Spinal Unit, Rookwood Hospital, Llandaff, Cardiff. *Telephone:* Cardiff 566281
Glasgow	Philips Hill Hospital, Nr. Glasgow. *Telephone:* 041–644 1144
Hexham	Hexham General Hospital, Hexham, Northumberland. *Telephone:* Hexham 2421
Musselburgh	Edenhall Hospital, Musselburgh, Midlothian. *Telephone:* 031–665 2546
Oswestry	The Midland Spinal Injuries Centre, Robert Jones & Agnes Hunt Orthopaedic Hospital, Oswestry, Salop. *Telephone:* Oswestry 5311
Sheffield	The Spinal Unit, Lodge Moor Hospital, Sheffield S10 4LH. *Telephone:* Sheffield 306555

Southport   The Spinal Unit,
                                   Promenade Hospital,
                                   Southport, Lancs.
                                   Telephone:
                                   Southport 5158

Wakefield   The Spinal Unit,
                                   Pinderfields General
                                   Hospital, Wakefield,
                                   Yorkshire.
                                    Telephone:
                                   Wakefield 0924

Eire   Our Lady of Lourdes
                                   Hospital,
                                   Dun Laoghaire, Eire.

ADDRESSES OF HER MAJESTY'S STATIONERY OFFICES

Atlantic House   Bankhead Avenue
Holborn Viaduct   Edinburgh, EH11 4AB
London, EC1P 1BN

Broadway   Ashton Vale Road
Chadderton, Oldham   Ashton
Lancs. OL9 9QH   Bristol, BS3 2HN

Sovereign House   Chichester House
Botolph Street   Chichester Street
Norwich, NR3 1DN   Belfast, BT1 4PS

ADDRESSES OF USEFUL ORGANIZATIONS IN THE UNITED STATES OF AMERICA AND CANADA

U.S.A.
National Paraplegia Foundation,
333N Michigan Avenue,
Chicago,
Illinois 60601.
Telephone (312) 346–4779

Paralyzed Veterans of America,
7315 Wisconsin Avenue, Suite 300W,
Washington D.C. 20014.
Telephone (301) 652–2135

Texas Institute for
Rehabilitation & Research,
1333 Moursund Avenue,
Houston,
Texas.

The Yellow Pages of the telephone directory will give the addresses of the divisional offices in each state for both the National Paraplegia Foundation and the Paralyzed Veterans of America. Both these organizations will supply a wide range of helpful literature as well as practical advice.

Canada
Canadian Paraplegic Association,
520 Sutherland Drive,
Toronto,
Ontario, M4G 3V9.

Index